THE SENSUAL BATH

STERLING and the distinctive Sterling logo are registered
trademarks of Sterling Publishing Co., Inc.

Library of Congress Cataloging-in-Publication Data Available

10 9 8 7 6 5 4 3 2 1

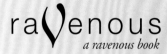

a ravenous book

Produced by Ravenous
An imprint of Hollan Publishing, Inc.
100 Cummings Center, Suite 125G
Beverly, MA 01915

© 2008 by Hollan Publishing, Inc.
Published by Sterling Publishing Co., Inc.
387 Park Avenue South, New York, NY 10016

Distributed in Canada by Sterling Publishing
c/o Canadian Manda Group, 165 Dufferin Street
Toronto, Ontario, Canada M6K 3H6
Distributed in the United Kingdom by GMC Distribution Services
Castle Place, 166 High Street, Lewes,
East Sussex, England BN7 1XU
Distributed in Australia by Capricorn Link (Australia) Pty. Ltd.
P.O. Box 704, Windsor, NSW 2756, Australia

Printed in Singapore
All rights reserved

Sterling ISBN-13: 978-1-4027-4933-9
        ISBN-10: 1-4027-4933-3

For information about custom editions, special sales, premium and
corporate purchases, please contact Sterling Special Sales Depart-
ment at 800-805-5489 or specialsales@sterlingpublishing.com.

Photography by Allan Penn
Cover and interior design by Carol Holtz/Holtz Design
Photo on page 24 by Roderick Chen/Jupiter Images
Photo on page 40 by Amy Neunsinger/Jupiter Images

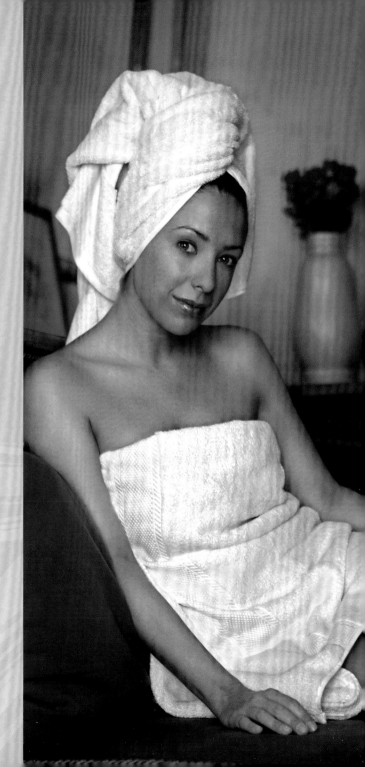

TAMAR LOVE

THE SENSUAL BATH

Soaking in Pleasure and Passion

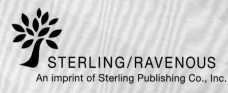

STERLING/RAVENOUS
An imprint of Sterling Publishing Co., Inc.

New York / London
www.sterlingpublishing.com

Contents

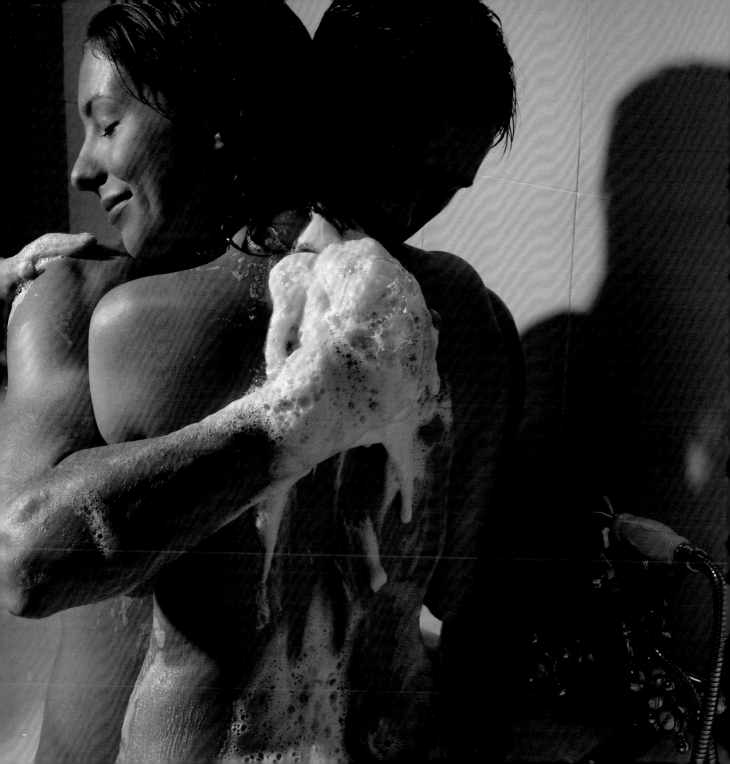

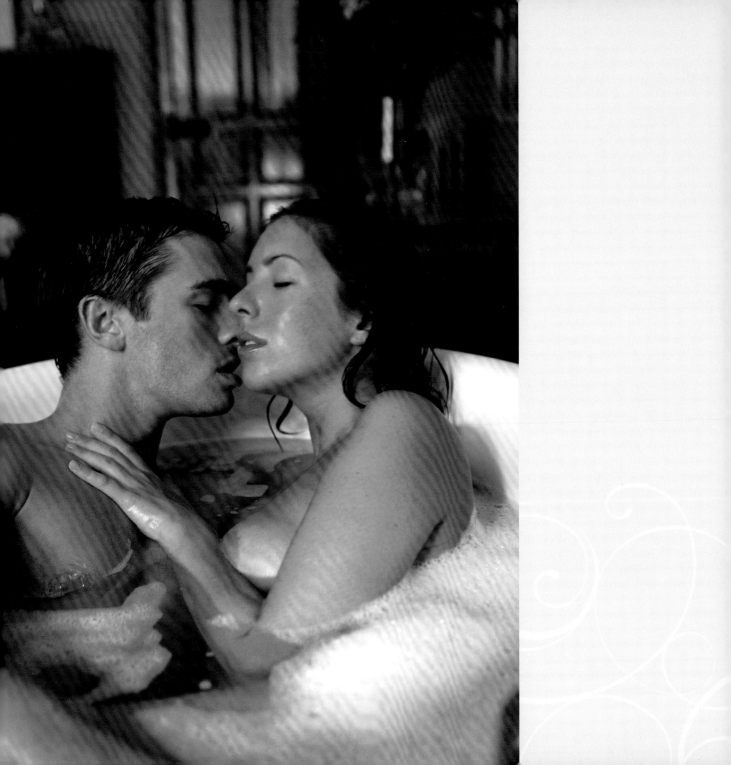

Introduction

WHILE WATER HAS BEEN used since antiquity as a symbol by which to express devotion and purity, its vitality, energy, and sensuality also make it highly erotic and arousing. Water can intensify touch, and wetness can be incredibly sexy. The warm, intimate nature of the bath makes it the perfect environment for celebrating sensuality. Light a few candles, fill the tub with water, slip out of your clothes and relax into a sensual bath. Drape a wet washcloth over your eyes and tune out the world for twenty minutes. If you prefer, invite your partner and celebrate your sensuality together—the bath is a superb locale for exploring the sexual possibilities of the sensual bath.

If you've never enjoyed a sensual bath, this book will help you explore a new form of sexual expression. If you have never bathed with your lover before, you have an exciting adventure ahead of you.

Tub-time Tips

Throughout *The Sensual Bath,* "Tub-time Tips" will share practical, sensual, and erotic bathing advice to ensure that you get the most out of your sensual bathing experience (and that includes more than just getting clean!).

The Alchemist

You'll also find lots of fun recipes in *The Sensual Bath,* instructions for making lotions and potions and other luscious delicacies. You don't have to be a chemist or culinary genius to make these recipes work, and you won't have to search for obscure ingredients. All the recipes in this book utilize only very basic kitchen skills, and the ingredients are all easily obtainable from online retailers, grocery stores, and natural food stores nationwide.

The first time you try a recipe, follow the directions carefully and test out the product before you use it. If you want to make alterations after that, start with small changes, like using different scents or flavorings. Use fresh ingredients, clean tools, and good common sense!

A Little Spice Is Nice

There's nothing wrong with sticking to the basics, but sometimes the occasion calls for a little something extra. When you want to turn up the heat, flip to the suggestion boxes you'll find throughout this book and learn how to "Spice It Up."

Personalizing Your Sensual Bath

After you experiment with the ideas in *The Sensual Bath,* feel free to recombine elements and create an experience that is unique to you. Bathing can be an intimate and erotic ritual, so it's essential that you create a sensual bath that is personal to you.

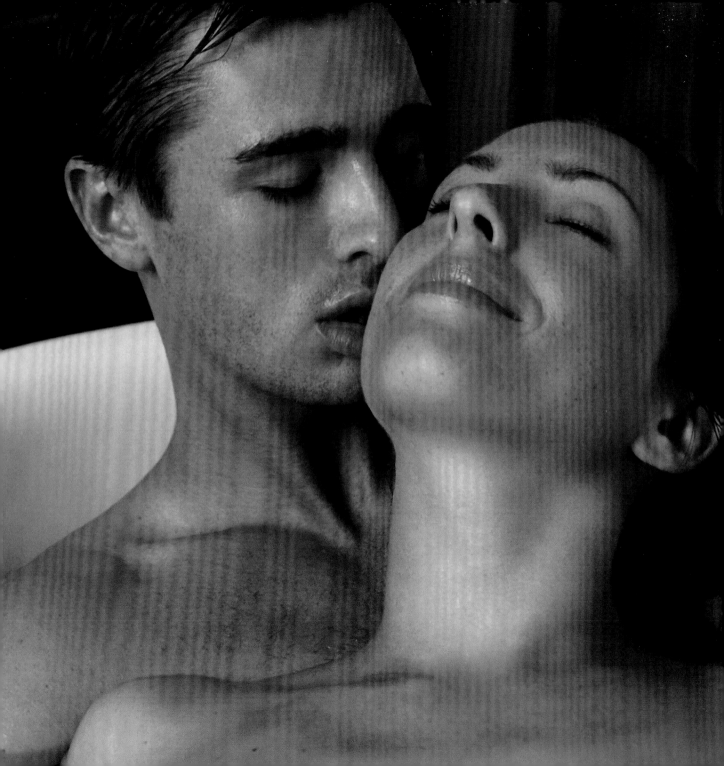

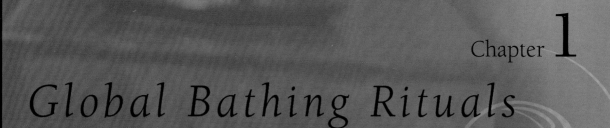

Chapter 1

Global Bathing Rituals

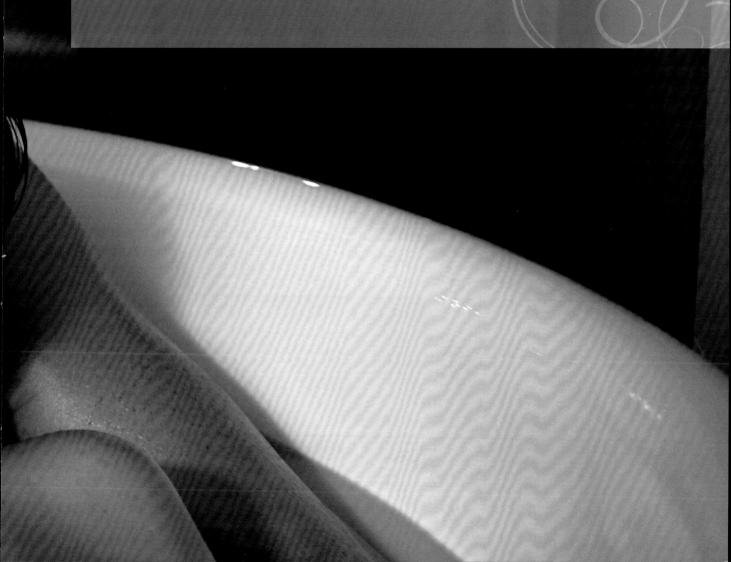

THE HISTORY OF LUXURIOUS BATHING

SINCE THE BEGINNING of recorded history, people all over the world have enjoyed the pleasures of a hot bath. The initial objective may have been cleansing oneself, but as various cultures developed over time, bathing often became ritualized, and enjoyed by the upper-class and religious sectors of society.

THE AFFLUENT EVOLVED BATHING into an art form, adding luxurious touches such as expansive bathing rooms and expensive soaps and lotions. Meanwhile, the priests and clerics incorporated cleansing into their religious rituals, exposing the common people to the sensual pleasure of bathing. Communal bathing and public bathhouses, which exist in different forms within almost every culture, became an essential part of the society. Eventually all the people, rich or poor, secular or religious, would come to find the same comforts in the bath: warm water to clean unkempt bodies, steam and massage to soothe sore muscles, and a nexus for social interaction.

Things aren't much different today. At the gym, we work out, talk with friends, and bathe in a communal locker room facility. At health spas, we gossip and relax, pampering our bodies while we rejuvenate our minds. We often use the ritual of bathing as a way to cleanse our bodies before we share them with another, incorporating sensual elements with roots in ancient cultures and faraway lands.

Ancient Egypt

One of the most advanced cultures in the ancient world, Egyptians regarded cleanliness as an important part of daily life. Most people cleansed themselves using a water basin at home; those fortunate enough to live near a river bathed there. Only the very wealthy had an entire room—or suite of rooms—devoted to bathing, as well as servants whose function was to pour clean water over their masters.

If no water was available, as is often the case in the desert, ancient Egyptians used perfumed oil to cleanse themselves, working the oil into their skin and using a sharp blade to scrape away hair and dirt. Although the process wasn't very sexy, it resulted in soft, smooth, perfumed skin, which has always been *very* sexy.

Ancient Egyptians made their linens from the flax plant, but more modern denizens of the desert land use an extralong staple cotton to produce the thick, luxurious towels we enjoy today. Oversized Egyptian cotton bath linens are ideal for drying off after a relaxing bath—nothing feels more luxe than plush Egyptian cotton on clean skin.

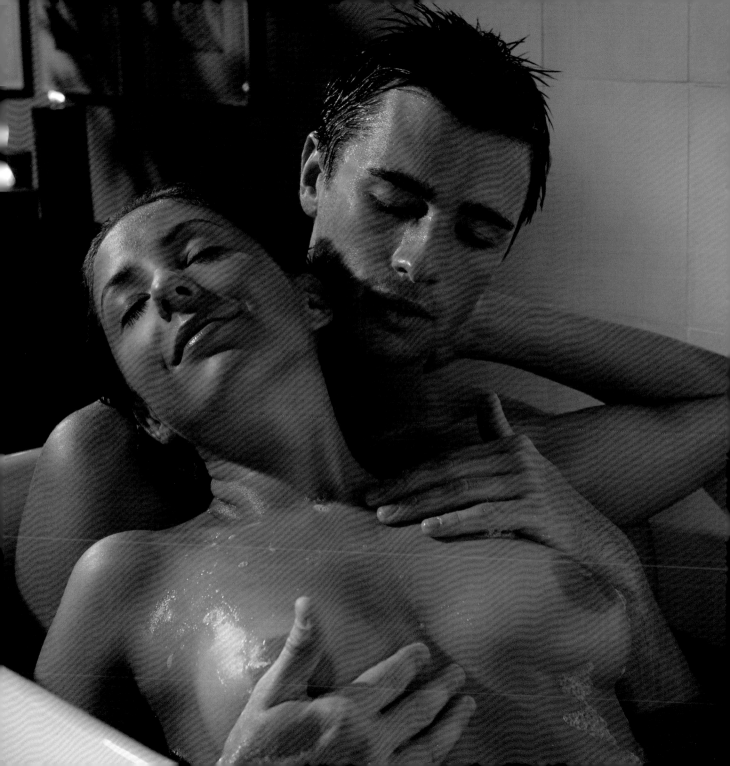

The Roman Empire

In a society ruled by a strict class system, bathing was the great equalizer in ancient Rome. Enjoyed daily by men and women of all stations in life, this leisure activity was a communal experience that usually occurred in public bathhouses.

The larger bathing houses were called *thermae*, while the smaller public houses (usually privately owned), known as *balneae*, were open to everyone except slaves and those too poor to afford even the very small admission fee. Some *thermae* had separate bathing rooms for men and women, while other facilities were open to women in the morning and men in the afternoon, usually around 2:00 p.m. Both men and women used *thermae* for much more than getting clean. Both sexes enjoyed the social aspects of communal bathing—sharing gossip, conducting affairs of state, and discussing business matters—as well as the opportunity for exercise, sport, and recreation.

Although the wealthy often had a room—or series of rooms—devoted entirely to their daily ablutions, they still visited public bathhouses, whose design, purpose, and usage resembled modern-day health spas and gyms. Upon arrival, bathers would remove their street clothes and shoes, storing them in the *apodyterium*—similar to today's locker room—before proceeding to the *palaestra,* the open courtyard, where the men practiced weight lifting, wrestling, ball playing, running, and other sports. Bathing took place in the *caldarium,* the area closest to the furnace room, whose function resembled today's sauna and locker room.

My boyfriend, Scott, and I have developed a modern version of the Roman bath. After work on Friday, we jog through Central Park, and then when we get home, we shower together and wash each other's bodies. When we're nice and clean, we slip into his oversized whirlpool tub to soak and massage each other's sore muscles. As we relax and shed the worries of the week, Scott and I reconnect—first mentally, and then physically, which is really the highlight of the ritual!

—*Amber, 28*

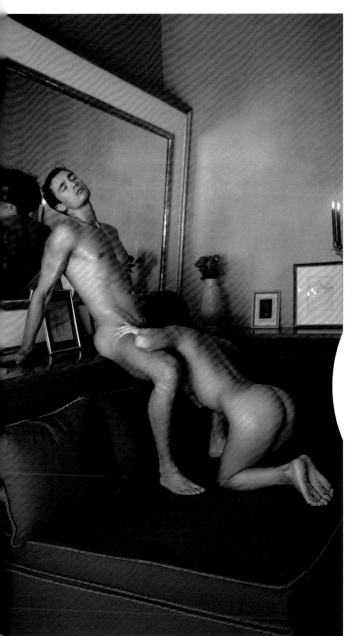

"Mixed bathing" between men and women was discouraged; in fact, the Emperor often forbade it, suggesting that even though bathhouses were places to bathe for cleanliness, people enjoyed getting "dirty"— engaging in sexual acts—there, too. A woman's reputation would be ruined if she were discovered bathing with a man not her husband, but the men openly enjoyed the attentions of male slaves and female prostitutes. Ancient Rome, birthplace of the aqueduct, the Republic, and the double standard!

Tub-time Tips

RIDING THE JET STREAM

We may owe the concept of the health spa to the ancient Romans, but the Jacuzzi tub is a purely modern invention. Either alone or with a partner, the Jacuzzi jets can be even more satisfying (and not just for cleansing!) than a handheld showerhead.

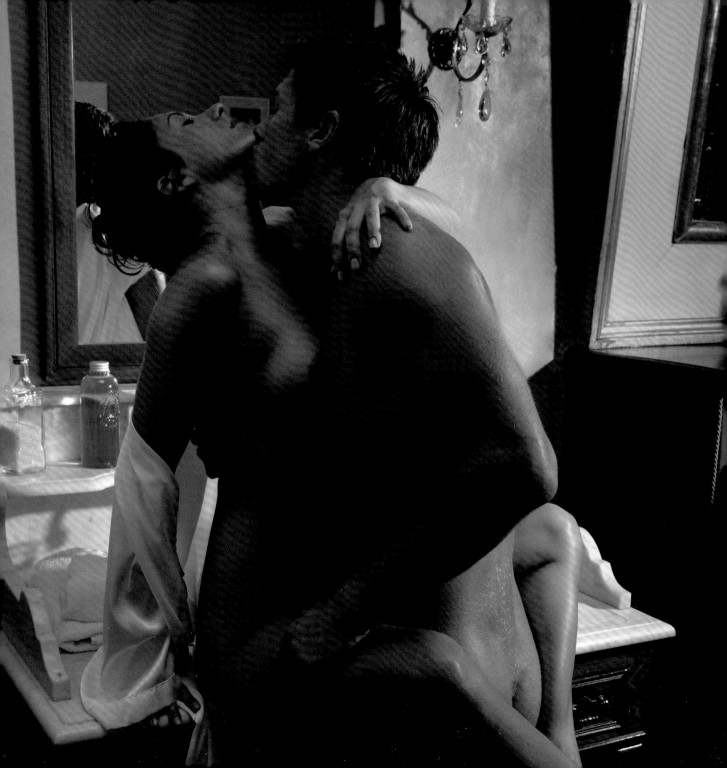

Japanese Baths

In Western culture, bathing is usually focused on washing away the day's grime. In Japanese culture, however, bathing is about much more than cleansing the body. A ritualized process with roots in Shintoism and Buddhism, the Japanese bath refreshes the body and mind and is thought to do the same to a person's spirit.

Ofuro, the Japanese hot bath, is often a communal experience dating back to the early years of Japan's history. Royal persons, monks, and the wealthy would often enjoy long, elaborate baths. As these baths became more popular, bathhouses for the common people were opened so that everyone could enjoy cleanliness of body and mind.

The primary difference between *ofuro* and the communal hot baths common to other cultures is that the Japanese cleanse themselves *before* they slip into the bath. In the United States, people run a bath and soak for a bit in what can quickly become a tub filled with dirty water. In Japanese culture, bathers thoroughly cleanse their bodies before they even step into the tub. This practice not only enables the bather to soak in deliciously clean water, but also allows multiple bathers to enjoy the same water without a soiled ring forming around the tub.

My wife and I share a ritual many people would find strange: we bathe before we bathe together. We're not clean freaks or anything like that—my wife is an ER nurse and I work construction, so getting clean before we touch each other is absolutely necessary.

Since we love soaking together in our oversized tub, we meet there after we've cleaned up in separate bathrooms. I've found that when she's already clean and relaxed, she's much more open to giving and receiving oral sex—which is always a welcome treat!

—Jason, 38

In traditional Japanese homes, the bathing area is usually separate from the toilet area and contains not only a bathtub, but also a tiled area resembling an open shower, equipped with a small stool, a bucket or pan of water, a handheld showerhead, and assorted bathing products, such as soap and shampoo. Before soaking in the tub, bathers first clean themselves thoroughly, cleansing and exfoliating their skin; shampooing and moisturizing their hair; and scrubbing their hands, feet, and nails. By the time the bather relaxes into a tub of hot, clean water, his or her body is already squeaky clean. The bath then becomes totally focused on relaxation of the body and refreshment of the mind.

Although *ofuro* is not traditionally a sexual experience, it is most certainly sensual: the clean, hot water relaxes the senses and opens the mind, serving as the perfect prelude to lovemaking. Easily adapted to Western needs, the communal tradition of *ofuro* can function as a practical way to build intimacy between partners, before or after sex.

Ofuro and the Sensual Bath

Even though your bathroom might be 100 percent Western, you can easily enjoy *ofuro* at home.

1. In your bedroom or dressing area, remove all clothing and jewelry. Enter your bathroom naked, equipped with a clean robe and a fresh pair of slippers.

2. Set a small, plastic stool in the dry tub or shower stall or sit on the edge of the tub. If you prefer, stand in the shower or tub.

3. Use the handheld showerhead to thoroughly wet your body and hair. Turn off the water and wash your body and hair, scrubbing yourself clean.

4. Rinse yourself, being sure to wash away all traces of dirt, soap, and shampoo; rinse the tub clean when you are done.

5. Run a fresh, hot bath, adding essential oils or bath salts, as you desire. If you have long hair, pin it up.

6. Ease into the hot water and enjoy a long soak that cleanses your mind and spirit. After your bath, slip into your clean robe and slippers.

The pre-bathing aspects of *ofuro* are traditionally experienced alone, but you and your partner might enjoy the intimacy of cleansing each other before you bathe together.

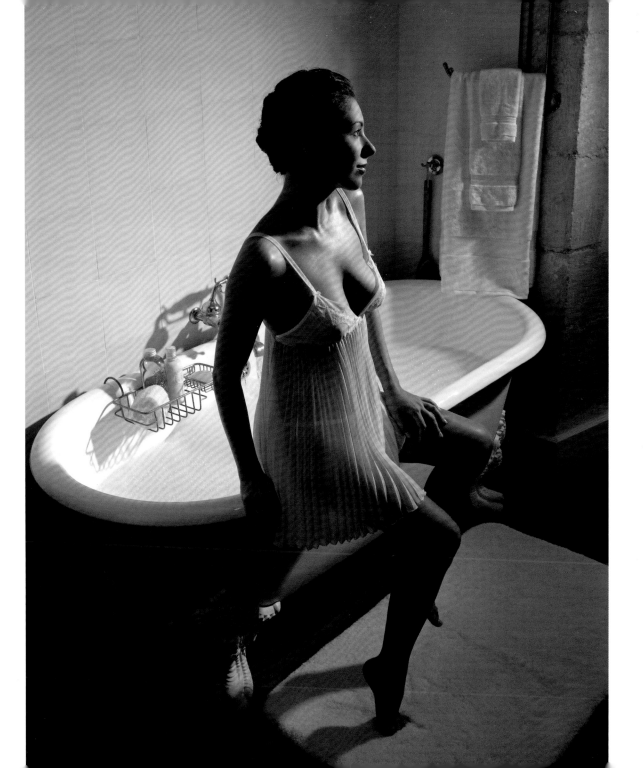

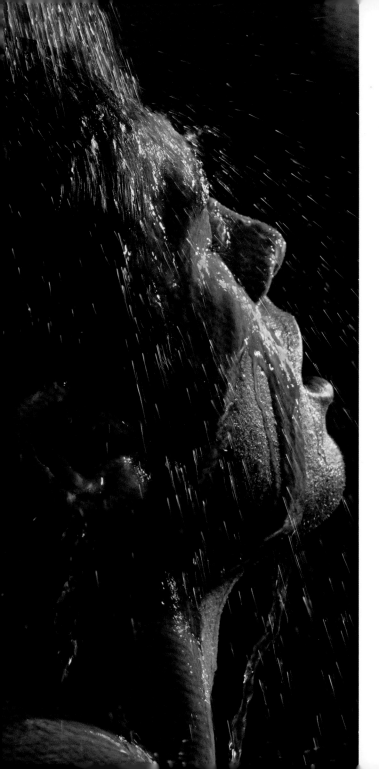

Turkish Baths

Predominantly Muslim, the Turks took the required bathing of their religion and culture and incorporated elements that were hedonistic and exotic, most notably steam, and created the tradition known as *hamam*.

The bathing ritual itself began with a relaxing sit in a warm room, heated by a continuous flow of hot, dry air. As the steam opened the bathers' pores, dirt and other toxins left the body. The bather could then move to a hot room—increased perspiration was thought to cleanse the internal organs, especially the lungs. After leaving the hot room, the bather would splash cold water on his face and body before enjoying a full-body wash and massage. The *hamam* ended with a few relaxing moments—or a pleasant afternoon—in the cooling-off room.

The men's *hamam* was a place for discussions of business or politics, but for women, the *hamam* was the center of society. Escorted by servants bearing delicacies of food and drink, the procession of ladies drew every eye as they moved from the harem to the *hamam*, where they would spend hours in the hot steam, the younger women giggling and comparing embroidered finery, while the older women gossiped and searched out possible matches for their sons.

History might not feel sexy, but it's essential for understanding why we do what we do. The tradition of bathing is no different: The sensual pleasures we enjoy today were first developed by ancient cultures. So the next time you step into a sauna, give a nod to the Turks, without whom you'd be sitting in a hot, steamless room.

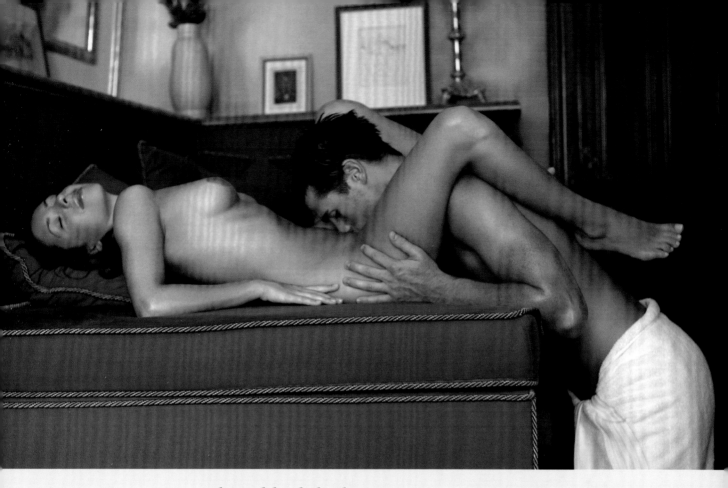

Edward had the best bathroom of any man I'd ever dated.
His shower was bigger than my walk-in closet, and the oversized
tub was equipped with whirlpool jets. He even had a small sauna,
just big enough for two. I'd never tried a sauna before, and I
was surprised at how much I enjoyed it. The hot air relaxed
every muscle in my body, but instead of feeling like Jell-o, I was
incredibly aroused. We rinsed off in the shower and then slipped
into the tub, where we made love for hours.

—Kendall, 24

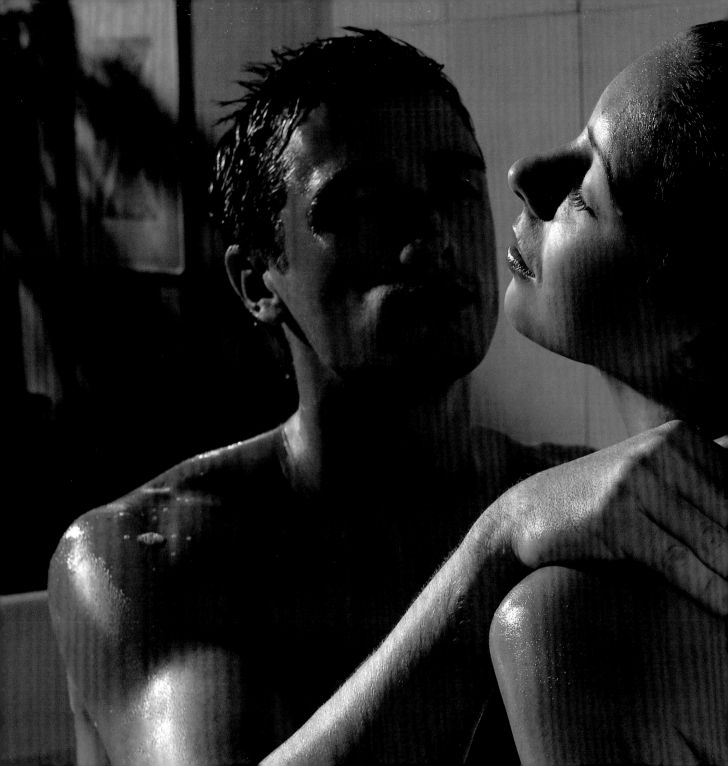

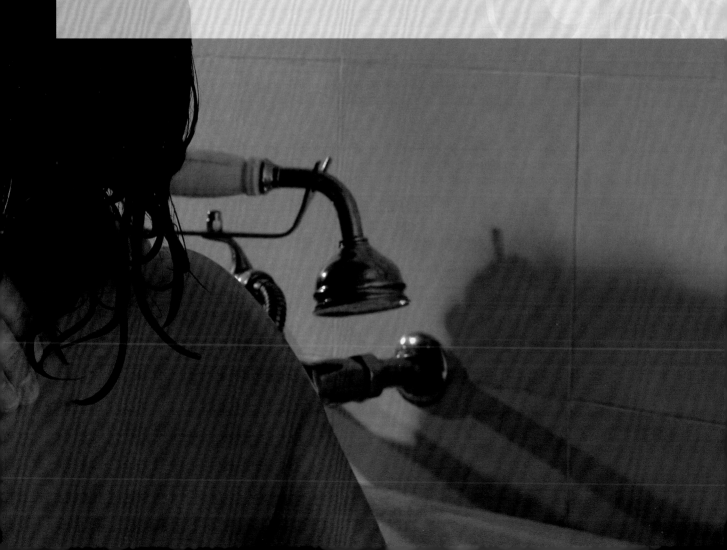

Chapter 2

The Physical Environment

BATHING AS AN ART FORM

ALTHOUGH DAILY BATHING has only been common for the last hundred years, the practice has already evolved into an art form, spawning a host of industries focused on supplying newer and better products for cleansing and pampering our bodies. Once only a place for tending to our bodies' basic functions, the bathroom is rapidly becoming the go-to place for nurturing our most basic human needs.

LUXURY BATHROOMS, once the purview of upscale hotels, are becoming commonplace, and homeowners everywhere are refitting their powder rooms with upgraded fixtures, stylish design elements, luxurious linens, and luxury spa products.

Even if you're renting, budgeting, or just not able to hire a professional design team to remodel your bathroom, you can still dress it up with a few simple touches.

Keep It Clean

It's not easy to feel sexy when you're soaking in a filthy tub—and who wants to make love in a bathroom with mildew on the walls and ceilings? Spend just one Saturday afternoon getting the bathroom really clean, and you'll never have to do it again.

Clear out all the cabinets and drawers, throwing away all the old toiletries and expired medications and getting rid of anything you don't use. Before you put anything away, clean the whole bathroom from top to bottom. Scour away mold, mildew, dirt, and soap scum. Launder all your linens, including shower or window curtains if you have them. As you put things back into drawers and cabinets, wipe off each item. When you're done, you'll have a space that is comfortable and pleasant.

Keeping the room clean is a lot easier than you think! Stow a small cleaning kit in the bathroom, and wipe up spills and messes as they happen. Use cleaning products designed to prevent soap-scum and mildew buildup, and remember to launder your towels once a week. Give the room a five-minute tidying once a week, cleaning the mirrors, countertops, toilet and sink.

If you don't have adequate storage in your bathroom, then pare down or get creative with organizational solutions. Relocate anything you can store elsewhere, such as your jewelry collection, the set of extra linens, or any warehouse-sized bundles of toilet paper.

When buying new items for the bathroom—anything from towels to tissue paper—aim for a simple, uniform look that will blend with your décor. Keep the counters bare and the towels neatly hung, and the bathroom will look clean and tidy, even when it's not. Remember, you'll be far more likely to indulge in a bath if you don't have to clean it first!

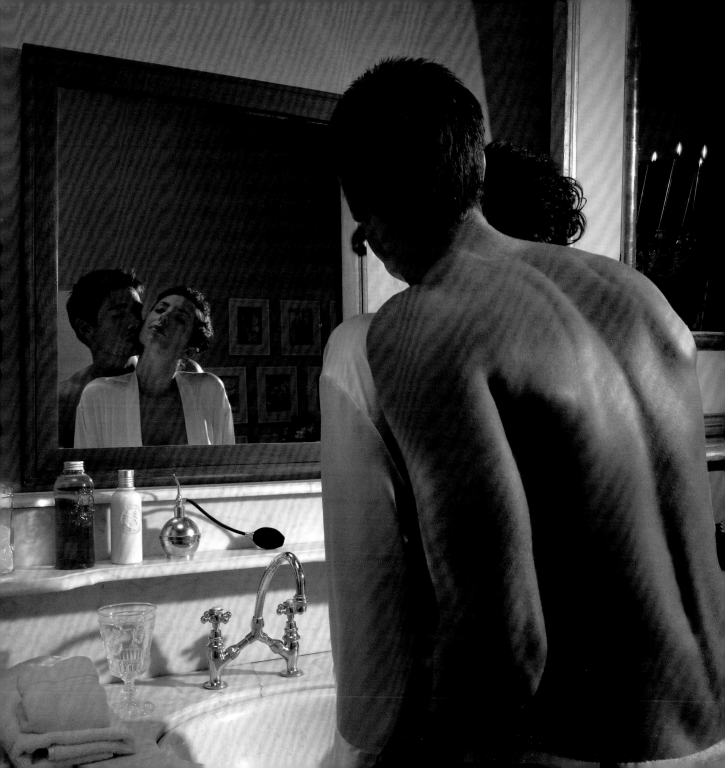

Make Easy Upgrades

Buying matching sink-top accessories is a good first step toward spa-style living, as is investing in a decent laundry hamper and trashcan. Even if you are renting, you can make surprisingly dramatic changes with a few easy, inexpensive projects.

Treat the Windows

Most bathrooms have only one window, if that. Swapping out the bargain-basement blinds for inexpensive wood or laminate blinds costs about $25; hanging new curtains costs even less. Both projects are easy enough for even amateurs to handle without mishap, and the results can redefine the entire room.

Refurbish the Fixtures

Simple bathroom hardware, like the toilet-paper holder, towel bars, shelves, and mirrors, are relatively inexpensive and very easy to switch out. If you shop sales, you should be able to get everything you need for $50 to $100, not a bad price when you consider the impact the change will make.

Tackle Larger Projects

If your bathroom is looking a little frayed around the edges, a few simple home-improvement projects can yield big results. If you are able to paint your bathroom, it's the single biggest change you can make. It's also quite simple to replace any missing grout around your tub, toilet, or sink. If you're limited to smaller projects, eradicate mildew, rust, or lime stains with the appropriate product from your local home-improvement store. Patch any holes in the walls with neutral-colored spackle.

Attend to the Details

Paying attention to the small details can make a tremendous difference, especially if you're on a tight budget, or have little time to invest. Use coordinating towels

Sparkling and clean, the bathroom is my personal spa, a tranquil oasis designed to soothe my aching body, ease my tired mind, and rejuvenate my spirit. The room is spacious and clean, filled with objects that are beautiful and useful, and I always have a stack of freshly laundered towels on a shelf. My spa helps me to relax, enabling me to be more present in my life, and a better lover to my husband.

—*Marisa, 35*

and matching countertop accessories, like the tissue-box cover, cup, soap holder, and lotion dispenser. Decant commonly used items—Q-tips, cotton squares, liquid soap, mouthwash—into attractive containers. Install matching switch-plate covers for your bathroom outlets and light switch, and buy matching knobs for all your bathroom drawers and cabinets.

Add Fresh Touches

If you aren't careful, the bathroom can start to smell odd after a while, a fusty smell that no amount of Lysol can eradicate. If you are fortunate to have a window, open it daily to air out unpleasant odors before they take over. If you have a fan, use it. If you're lacking any means to circulate the air, at least make sure you leave the bathroom door open after you shower or bathe, so that the steam can evaporate before the moisture has a chance to stink up the room. Natural light, live plants, and fresh, clean towels are also great room refreshers.

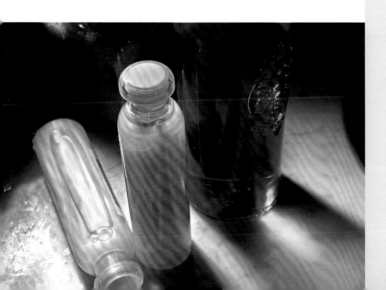

Stay Well Stocked

When you're relaxing into your sensual bath, you don't want to be caught short on shampoo (or lube!). Reaching for a needed product and coming up empty can really kill the mood, so keep your bathroom well stocked.

As you buy new bath supplies, get two of everything. One item gets used right away, and the other goes in the bathroom cabinet. When you run out of the product you're using—conditioner, shaving gel, bubble bath—you'll always have a backup on hand. Just remember to get a replacement and stick it back in the cabinet for next time.

Tub-time Tips

IT'S EASY BEING GREEN
Houseplants not only do an amazing job of adding style to any room, but also clean the air and make it easier to breathe. Plants are affordable and are simple to care for if you select plants that thrive in humidity and indirect sunlight, such as ferns, philodendrons, and pothos.

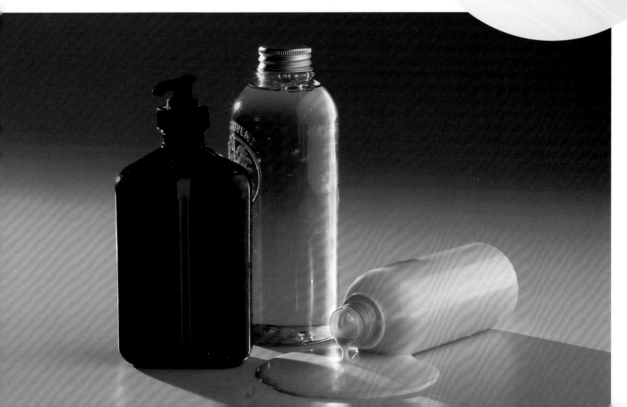

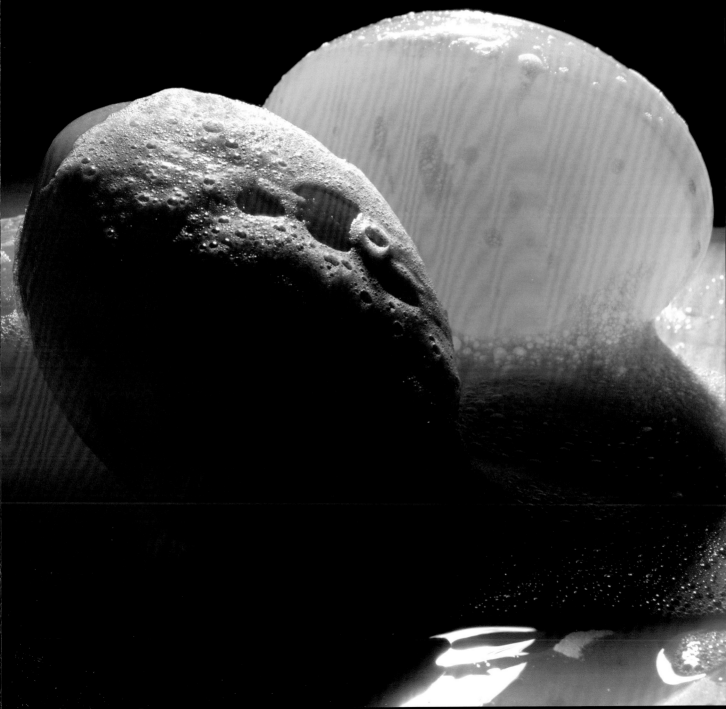

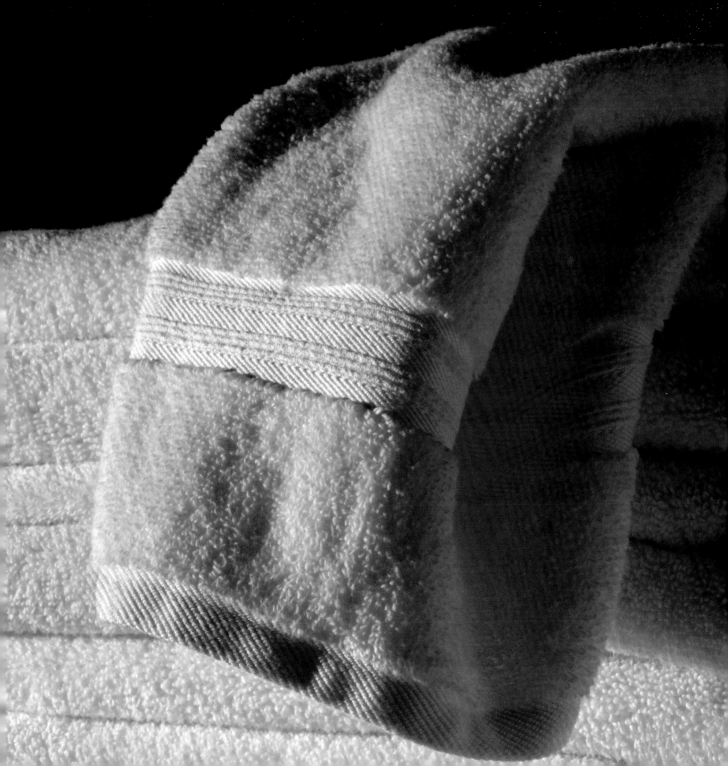

LITTLE LUXURIES

ONCE THE PHYSICAL environment of the bathroom begins to resemble a spa, it's time to upgrade the linens and bath products you use. Select toiletries and bath products with pleasing packaging and fragrances. You might be fifty cents poorer, but you'll enjoy the lavender-scented bath oil in the pretty bottle every time you look at it.

Once you begin to focus on the luxurious little extras that differentiate everyday bathing from sensual bathing, you may find that you're developing a taste for finer things, at least in the bath. Fortunately, homemade bath products are inexpensive and easy to make, and luxe linens can be purchased for mere dollars if you don't mind doing a little detective work.

Choosing Plush Linens

When it comes to sumptuous creature comforts, nothing beats 100 percent cotton towels, preferably made of super-soft Turkish or Egyptian cotton. Soft, thick, and durable, quality bath linens will last longer and wear better than discount versions, which means they're a better value in the long run.

Regular-sized bath towels will get you dry, but they won't surround your body in plush luxury like a bath sheet. Larger in size by about 50 percent, bath sheets are big enough to dry your body and hair, and then serve as a modest sarong after bathing. You'll want at least one bath sheet per person, as well as hand towels and washcloths. Sateen finishes might be pretty, but they aren't very absorbent, nor are towels with short,

tight weaves. For maximum hedonistic pleasure, select a thick towel with a soft, open weave.

Wash quality linens in cold water and dry on low heat. Don't use liquid fabric softener. If your towels become stiff after repeated washings, add a cup of white vinegar to the wash water. If you care for your bath linens properly, they can last for years, making them a worthwhile investment for anyone who enjoys the pleasures of the bath.

Using Luxe Bath Products

Although soap and water are quite sufficient for getting clean, you'll want something a little more extravagant for your sensual bath. Whether you purchase your bath products or make your own, take the time to select fragrances and textures that will enhance your experience.

Bubble Bath

Bubble bath does a few different things: It softens the bathwater with soapy bubbles, adds fragrance and moisturizing agents, and irritates the skin if used too often. Enjoy your bubble bath, but do so infrequently. If you have sensitive skin, make your own bubble bath or look for formulas that use natural ingredients. Otherwise, don't bother to spend a lot of money on bubble bath; like hand soap, it doesn't really improve with fancier ingredients.

If you decide to make your own bubble bath, you'll find all the ingredients you need at your local grocery and natural food stores. The recipe is almost universal: a mixture of purified water, liquid glycerin, and castile soap is the base to which you can add different combinations of essential oils.

Bath Oil

Another aromatic water-softener, bath oil is superior to bubble bath because it doesn't contain any dehydrating soap bubbles to irritate sensitive flesh. Only use bubble bath sparingly, but feel free to use bath oil whenever you bathe.

Although any kind of body oil, even massage oil, will do an OK job of enhancing your bathwater, bath oils specifically formulated for bath use will last longer and hold fragrance a bit better. Purchase quality bath oils in drugstores and bath stores, or make your own blends at home.

Bath Salts

Perhaps the best water-softener, bath salts are inexpensive to purchase and simple to make. Add a handful to your bathwater to soften your skin. Bath salts are also great for soaking during a pedicure.

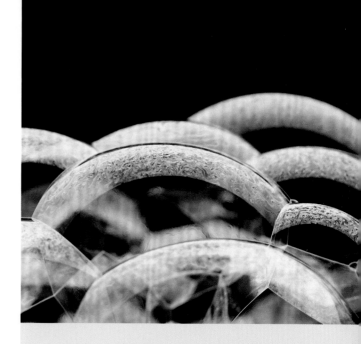

Romantic Interlude

A rich blend of sweet and floral scents gives this simple bubble bath a sensual fragrance.

1 quart (950 ml) distilled or boiled water
4 ounces (120 ml) liquid castile soap
4 ounces (120 ml) liquid glycerin
7 drops bergamot essential oil
7 drops jasmine essential oil
3 drops vanilla essential oil
3 drops ylang-ylang essential oil
3 drops rose essential oil (optional)

Add the liquid glycerin and castile soap to bath water. Mix well. Add essential oils. Rose oil can be expensive, so you may wish to omit it and increase the jasmine.

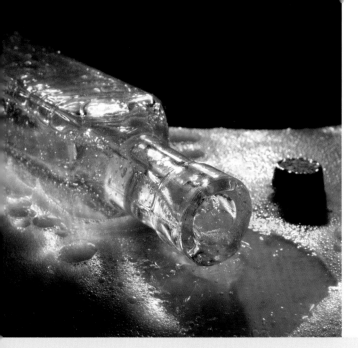

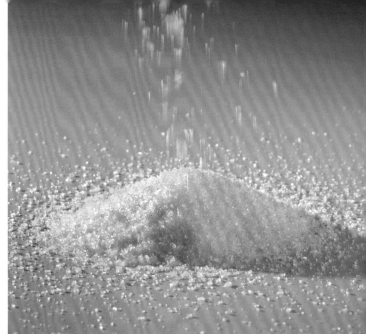

Basic Bath Oil

Creating beautiful, aromatic bath oils really could not be simpler. Sweet almond oil, available at any natural food, health, or bath store, is the base for your own selection of dried herbs and essential oils.

8 ounces (240 ml) sweet almond oil
1 tablespoon (15 ml) dried lavender, chamomile, or other herbal flowers
5 drops essential oils

Place herbal flowers into the bottom of a clean, dry, glass bottle, and then fill it with almond oil. Add a few drops of your favorite essential oils, cork tightly and shake gently to blend.

Basic Bath Salts

A longtime staple of elementary school craft classes, bath salts are just as easy for adults to make. Uncolored salts work just as well, but a little food coloring adds a pretty tint. Consult your elementary school color wheel for color ideas.

2 cups (600 g) Epsom salt
15 drops essential oils
2 to 3 drops food coloring (optional)

Place Epsom salt in a nonporous bowl and add essential oils. Mix with a fork to distribute evenly. If desired, add food coloring and mix well.

Accessorizing Well

As the bath connoisseur knows, a few well-chosen accessories can exponentially enhance the bathing experience. Don't load up your shower caddy with excessive accessories; select a few tools that best suit your needs.

Exfoliating Tools

The sensitive skin on your face and throat requires TLC, but the rest of you will respond to a hearty scrubbing with an exfoliating tool. Designed to remove dead cells and expose healthy, glowing skin, exfoliating tools have come a long way from the days of the wooden back brush. Choose from natural or synthetic loofahs in a variety of shapes and designs, or opt for a plain-Jane scrubby, available at any drug store. Use a washcloth to gently exfoliate more delicate regions, like the skin on your breasts and neck.

Feet and nails need cleaning, too, and there's no better place than the shower or bath. After you've spent a few minutes in the water, which will soften the tough skin on your feet and nails, use a nail brush to scrub your toenails and fingernails, cleaning under the nail and sloughing away dead skin on the cuticles. Use a pumice stone or Swedish file, available at drug and grocery stores, to smooth out calluses.

Sponges

An essential component of the essential sensual bath, a large bath sponge is perfect for squeezing warm water over exposed skin, be it your own or the back of a bathing partner. Natural sea sponges are organic alternatives to synthetic sponges, are relatively inexpensive, and look particularly attractive as part of your bathroom décor.

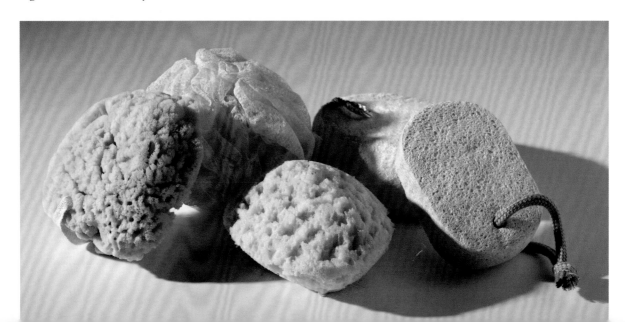

Bath Pillows

An increasingly popular accessory in tubs worldwide, bath pillows are small, inflatable, terry cloth–covered, waterproof pillows, usually equipped with suction cups to hold it in place against the tub wall. If you're a regular bather, a bath pillow is a necessity, especially if you read in the tub. A warm, wet washcloth will also provide a buffer against the cold porcelain, but it doesn't have the cushioning qualities of a cozy bath pillow.

Spice It Up

INSTANT ERGONOMICS

In a pinch, an inflatable bath pillow can work nicely as an ergonomic aid when you're getting down and dirty in the tub! The inflatable pillow helps counteract buoyancy and position your parts where they need to be for optimal penetration. Deflated, the pillow is a nifty makeshift tub mat, cushioning your bottom during sex, either solo or with a partner. Partially inflated, a bath pillow will even work as a kneepad while giving oral sex—just keep things brief lest you pop your prop mid-delivery.

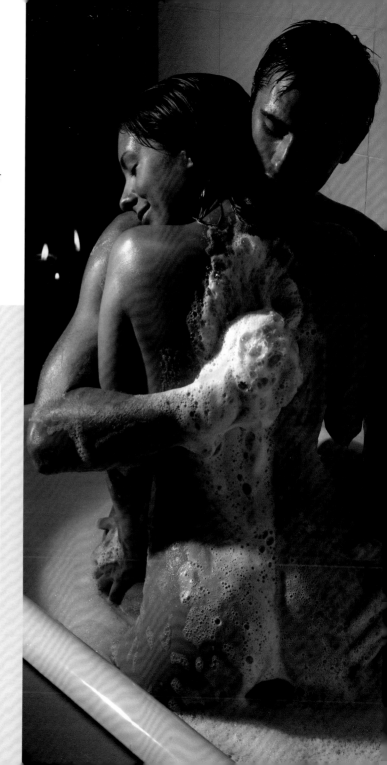

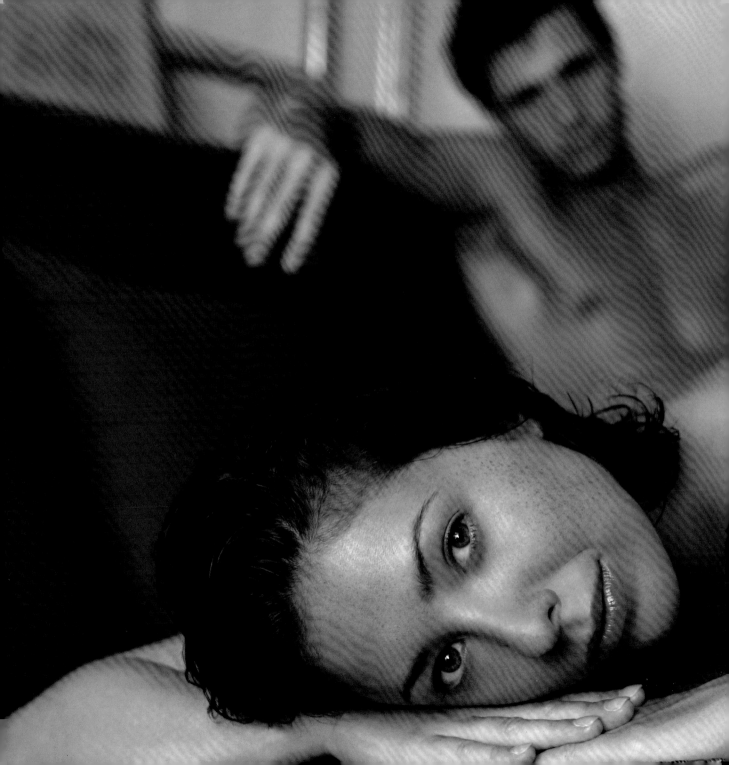

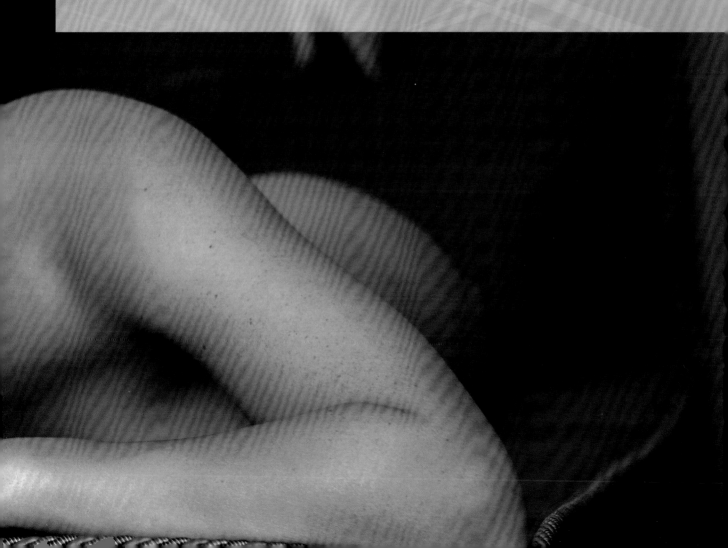

Chapter 3

The Sensual Environment

YOUR STEAMY SURROUNDINGS

THE WORD "SENSUAL" is not only a synonym for sexy, but also means appealing to the five senses: sight, sound, smell, touch, and taste. Although you'll certainly want to explore the sexy side of sensual bathing, take the time to stimulate *all* your senses. You'll enjoy a heightened state of arousal as your body and mind unite to experience complete sensual pleasure.

AS YOU PREPARE YOUR BATHROOM, be sure to balance your efforts equally with all five senses. Your objective is to create a harmonious union of sensual experiences; no one element should overpower the others.

Sight

Most people rely heavily on the sense of sight to direct their mood, especially where sex is concerned. Bright colors and cheerful lighting are nice in the kitchen, but rich colors and low ambient lighting are more conducive to sensuality.

Not everyone is able—or willing—to remodel their family bathroom into a powder room of erotic ecstasy. Fortunately, it only takes a few minutes to clear the clutter and set the scene for romance.

Background

Start with a clean bathroom. Empty the trash, wipe out the sink, and toss all the dirty laundry into the hamper. Even if it means you have to sweep everything into a drawer, remove all signs that anyone ever uses the room for anything other than sensual bathing. Once your background is prepped, you can personalize your sensual space with lighting and accessories.

Lighting

Most bathroom lighting is unpleasantly bright, suitable more for putting on makeup than playing with sex toys. Consider installing a dimmer switch—it's easier than you think—or keep a couple of lower-wattage bulbs handy for special occasions. Unless you are still in college, avoid choosing red or black-light bulbs.

If altering the lighting isn't an option, turn it off completely and fill the bathroom with candles. Not only will dozens of flickering flames give you enough illumination to read by, but they will also fill the room with warm, soft, romantic light.

Accessories

Accessorize your sensual space with items that appeal to your personal sense of beauty—a vase of fresh-cut flowers, a bowl of ripe fruit, beautifully packaged bath products. Even if you plan to read, your eyes will invariably wander off, so give yourself something pleasant to look at while you soak, even if it's something as simple as a stack of freshly laundered bath towels.

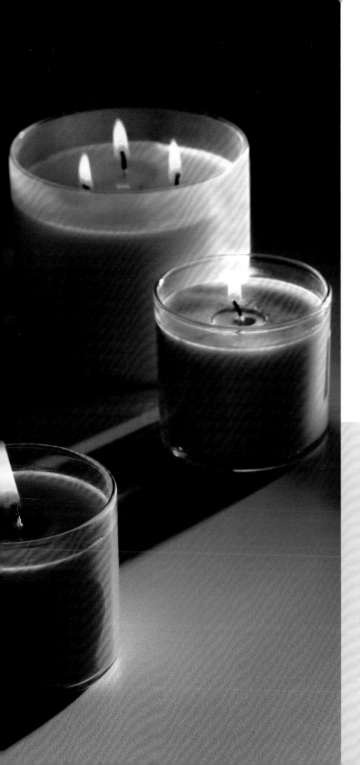

Smell

Although starting with a clean bathroom is an absolute necessity when you're planning to spend any amount of time in there, if you're drawing a sensual bath, you'll want to do more than just give the toilet a quick scrub.

Since the concept of aromatherapy exploded onto the Western market several decades ago, consumers have been deluged with scented everything: room spray, bath products, body lotion, even toilet paper and facial tissue. Too many conflicting odors can spoil a sensual mood, so prepare the room carefully. Don't overdo any one scent or scented product; instead, use essential oils to layer the room with scent.

Spice It Up

DRAMATIC STAGE DRESSING

If you hate your bathroom but don't have the time or funds to remodel, construct a temporary fix that will add drama to your sensual bathing experience. Drape the walls with high-end shower curtains or rich, gauzy fabric, using thumbtacks to secure it to the walls. Think of your fabric-covered walls as the backdrop for your sensual play.

Aromatherapy

The principles of aromatherapy focus on the therapeutic effects of essential oils on the mind, body, and spirit. Available at natural food stores and upscale grocery stores, essential oils are extracted from flowers, fruit, leaves, bark, and roots of plants and trees. A single drop produces intense effects, so even though these oils can be expensive, they last a long time, provided you keep them tightly bottled and stored in a dark, cool place.

Essential oils are extremely versatile. Try a few drops in your favorite unscented body lotion or bath oil, or add a few drops directly to bathwater. Blend a few of your favorite oils in an oil burner or diffuser. Add a drop to a hot, wet washcloth and drape it over your forehead while you soak. Invest in quality soy candles infused with essential oils; they'll burn longer and cleaner.

When thinking about which oils to try, consider more than just scent. Each oil has specific properties that interact differently with the body and mind.

Tub-time Tips

BURNING INCENSE

Incense not only makes the room smell better, but also affects our mental and physical states of being. Coordinate incense and bath scents by incorporating layers of the same scent, or burn a complementary fragrance to add depth to your olfactory ambiance.

BASIL—Although basil might seem more suited to the kitchen, the crisp, earthy scent is thought to increase sex drive, stimulate the senses, and calm an anxious mind.

BERGAMOT—Derived from the skin of a Moroccan cousin to the bitter orange, bergamot is a fresh-smelling, lightly floral citrus aroma that is said to refresh the senses, uplift the spirit, and prime lovers for deepening their bond.

CEDARWOOD—Thought to calm an anxious partner, cedarwood is a staple for anyone who uses essential oils in the bath. The fragrantly woody aroma of cedarwood is the base for many types of incense and oil blends.

CINNAMON—Cinnamon essential oil smells just like its culinary counterpart: exotic and spicy. In addition to being a pleasantly familiar scent, cinnamon is thought to soothe fatigue and revive the senses.

CITRUS—Although citrus essential oils have a more limited shelf life, lemon and orange essential oils are lovely added to bathwater and well worth buying frequently, especially since they are said to inspire playfulness and revive flagging relationships.

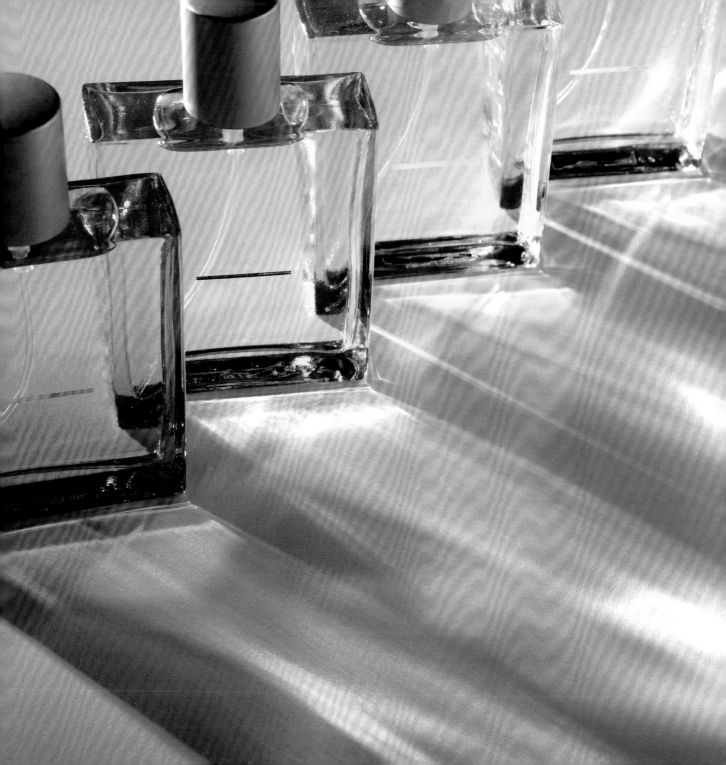

CLARY SAGE—This fresh, spicy, herbal aroma relaxes the body and has a calming effect on the mind. Clary sage has a mild euphoric effect and is thought to lower inhibitions and inspire more sensual behavior.

FRANKINCENSE—A fresh, balsamic, slightly lemony scent with fruity undertones, frankincense is thought to aid concentration by focusing and centering the emotions. Traditionally used in mediation and spiritual-growth practices, frankincense is commonly blended with lemon or orange essential oils.

GERANIUM—Thought to be beneficial for the reproductive organs, geranium oil is intensely floral. The sweet scent acts as a restorative, relaxing the body while strengthening the spirit. Commonly blended with rose essential oil, geranium alleviates depression.

LAVENDER—Possibly one of the most commonly used essential oils, lavender has a multitude of uses, from soothing anger and nervous tension to calming the mind and balancing the emotions. The earthy, richly floral aroma blends well with mint and clary sage.

JASMINE—Thought to be an aphrodisiac for hundreds of years, jasmine has the reputation for treating impotence and lowering inhibitions. Another essential oil staple, jasmine smells like the flower: sweet, heady, intense, exotic, and slightly fruity.

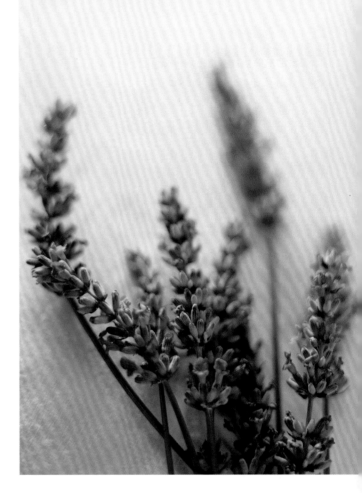

PATCHOULI—Despite its unfortunate association with unwashed hippies, patchouli remains one of the most popular and widely used essential oils. The heavy, musky, spicy, and intensely woody aroma penetrates the senses and clears the mind. Thought for centuries to have aphrodisiac qualities, patchouli mixes especially well with sandalwood.

PEPPERMINT—Minty and bracing, peppermint essential oil stimulates the senses and soothes a nervous stomach, making it a good choice for healing baths. The familiar sent of peppermint can also calm a nervous mind, and the sweet, crisp smell blends well with other oils, particularly lavender.

ROSE—Extremely effective at combating stress and exhaustion, the sweet, floral fragrance of rose oil is the ultimate in romance. In addition to being a mood enhancer, rose oil is also rumored to be an aphrodisiac. Blends well with geranium.

SANDALWOOD—Almost as well known as patchouli, sandalwood has a rich, warm, woody aroma that is oddly delicate. Thought to unite spiritual and sensual essences, sandalwood is wonderfully relaxing and blends well with other oils, especially patchouli and ylang-ylang.

YLANG-YLANG—Another aphrodisiac essential oil, ylang-ylang is sweetly floral, an intensely sensual scent that increases sex drive, lowers inhibitions, and promotes the feeling of well-being.

DON'T OVERWHELM THE SENSES with a confusion of aromas. You may prefer to stick with one fragrance group—floral, fruity, musky, or woody—using a citrus room spray, orange-bergamot bath oil, lemony body lotion, and a grapefruit scented candle. You might also enjoy combining complementary fragrances to create a complex sensual ambiance, perhaps sandalwood incense, patchouli body soap, a ylang-ylang scented candle. Keep it simple: Don't burn three kinds of incense and four different scented candles. The room's ambience should be warm and inviting, its fragrance pleasing and somewhat subtle. As with all five senses, keep your sense of smell balanced so that it doesn't overpower you. Each sense should add equally to your experience.

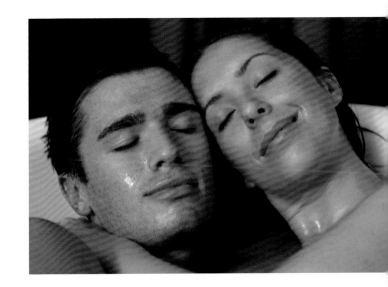

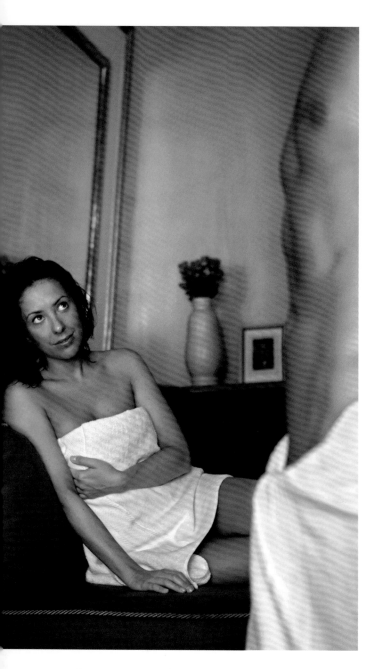

Recipes for a Sensual Bath

Just as you appeal to the five senses with flowers, rich creams, tasty treats, beautiful décor, and soothing sounds, your bathwater should also appeal to you sensually. Use water that is only a degree or two warmer than your body; hotter water can unpleasantly dehydrate you. Add a few drops of baby oil to soften the water.

Lavender, citrus, and geranium oils make good bases for romance. A good collection of essential oils will also include a couple of exotic scents, such as cinnamon, peppermint, and sandalwood. Try a few different scents to see what appeals to you best, or try one of these essential oil "recipes."

Tranquility

A deep, fragrant blend, this bath will soothe your body.

    2 drops lavender
    2 drops bergamot
    2 drops cedarwood

Energy

This zesty blend energizes the body and mind.

    3 drops rosemary
    2 drops lemon
    2 drops frankincense

Happiness

Playful and fun, this blend brings out the inner child.

    1 drop geranium
    2 drops frankincense
    2 drops orange

Romance

This fragrant blend is perfect for romantic evenings.

3 drops ylang-ylang

2 drops jasmine

1 drop sandalwood

1 drop patchouli

Seduction

A sweet, heady mix, this oil blend is light and sexy on the surface, but passionate and exotic underneath.

4 drops sandalwood

1 drop ylang-ylang

1 drop clary sage

1 drop rose

Gentle Love

This complex, multilayered scent smells like making love in the rain.

4 drops ylang-ylang

1 drop patchouli

1 drop black pepper

2 drops clary sage

1 drop neroli

1 drop rose

1 drop jasmine

Sensual Ecstasy

Richly floral, this blend is the perfect choice for a night of wild, passionate sex.

2 drops lavender

2 drops ylang-ylang

1 drop basil

1 drop geranium

1 drop bergamot

THE PLANNER IN YOU might be tempted to mix up a big batch of a particular bath recipe for use over time, but the oils need to remain in their pure form until you're ready to use them, so make each bath recipe only as you use it.

I used to think aromatherapy was just some New Age thing, but when a friend gave me a set of essential oils as a housewarming gift, I decided to give them a try. I tried a few combinations before settling on one that works: peppermint, lavender, and sandalwood. I like how the bathwater feels and smells, it makes my skin feel smooth, and the blend clears my mind after a long day.

—Bradley, 34

Hearing

The sounds of nature or the trickle of running water can be wonderfully relaxing, as can the sound of silence. Many people need little else to appease their need for sound stimulus during a sensual bath. However, a little mood music can do wonders for the ambiance, especially if you're bathing with your lover.

Your bathroom's acoustics will amplify loud noise, so stick with the basics: jazz, classical, soft rock, R&B. If your goal is to create a dramatic experience, you can experiment with house music, rock, rap, and even heavy metal, as long as everyone is amenable. Pop a few CDs in the changer or program your MP3 player with at least an hour's worth of music. You may need to change the song or adjust the volume while you're bathing, so keep the remote handy.

Music should enhance your bathing experience, not overwhelm it. Keep the volume low enough so that you and your partner can still converse easily; you can always turn it up when things get hot and heavy.

Everyone has their own favorite "bedroom" music—CDs they turn to when planning a romantic evening in the boudoir. Give the same attention to your sensual bath setup with one of the ambient albums listed on page 41.

Be sure to rotate your bathing music so the sound doesn't go stale. Introducing a new album to your ritual can be as exciting as trying a new position. If you make a mix CD, try to match your body's natural rhythms. Start off with slow songs that get you in the mood, ramp up to more feverish tunes, and throw in some gentle afterglow music for the very end.

For Valentine's Day, I made my girlfriend a mix CD to put on when we're making love in the shower. The music starts with smooth jazz and R&B, getting us both in the mood, and then progresses to hard, fast rock. The CD ends with a few love songs, which play after we've both climaxed. It's an erotic and sensual bathing experience, to say the least!

—Paul, 26

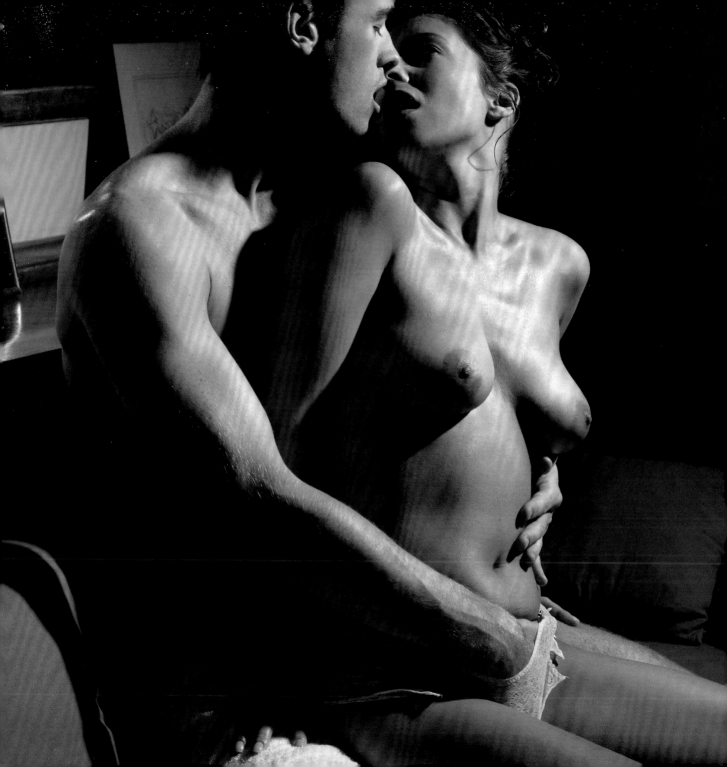

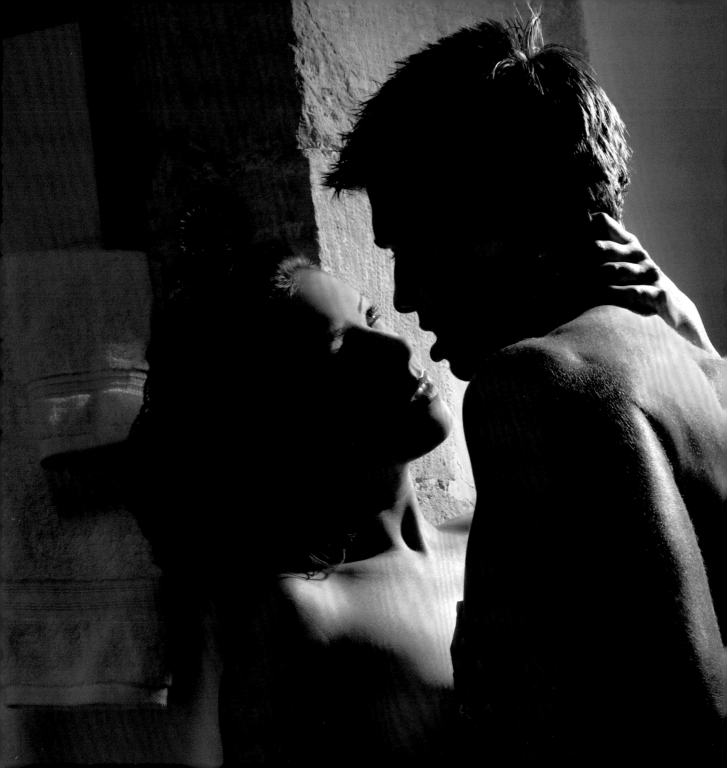

Sensual Sounds

Love Deluxe, Sade
The warm, honeyed voice of Sade crooning smooth jazz is the perfect aural backdrop for any kind of sensual bath, especially romantic partner bathing.

The Space Between Us, Craig Armstrong
From *William Shakespeare's Romeo + Juliet* composer Craig Armstrong, this CD is the musical equivalent of passionate sex, from foreplay to intercourse to climax to afterglow. Enjoy alone or with a partner.

Yo-Yo Ma Plays Ennio Morricone
Romantic without being schmaltzy, classic cellist Yo-Yo Ma interprets the moving, passionate music of film composer Ennio Morricone. Perfect for solo experiences, this CD will rouse your spirit and revive your mind.

Fumbling Towards Ecstasy, Sarah McLachlan——The folk-rock superstar's seminal album is moody and passionate, a beautiful accompaniment for women bathing alone.

Passion, Peter Gabriel
Still the most exotic lovemaking CD ever, Peter Gabriel's *The Last Temptation of Christ* soundtrack captures deeply sensual Middle Eastern and African sounds. Perfect for any bathing experience, alone or with a partner.

Blue Lines, Massive Attack
The deep beats, melodic vocals, and soulful ambiance of this classic house CD make it a perfect choice for men bathing together or alone.

Come Away with Me, Norah Jones
Nothing calms the spirit like Norah Jones's sleepy jazz tunes. This album is sure to slow things down (in a good way) and help you enjoy a long, sexy soak.

Cantos de Amor, Gipsy Kings
The Flamenco-style guitar and passionate vocals of this album will make bath time feel like an exotic getaway. It's best to enjoy this little "vacation" with a partner.

Touch

Perhaps the most sensual of the five, our sense of touch is often woefully overlooked—after all, skin is our largest, most sensitive organ. Take a few moments to tantalize yourselves with luxurious sensation; the payoff is total immersion in sensual pleasure.

Sensual caressing—courtesy of yourself or a partner—is only the most obvious way to appeal to your sense of touch. It's easy to overlook bathwater as a touch stimulus, but during a sensual bath, water is the one thing that touches every part of your skin. Plain water doesn't feel like much, but water softened with bath oil or salts feels luxuriant against the skin, as do silk pajamas or lingerie or a thick, plush robe.

Spice It Up

INSTANT ERGONOMICS

The extremes of heat and cold can be highly erotic, especially when combined with fantasy play. Try blindfolding your partner and dripping hot wax on your lover's belly, thighs, nipples, or buttocks. Follow up the burst of heat with the gentle touch of an ice cube.

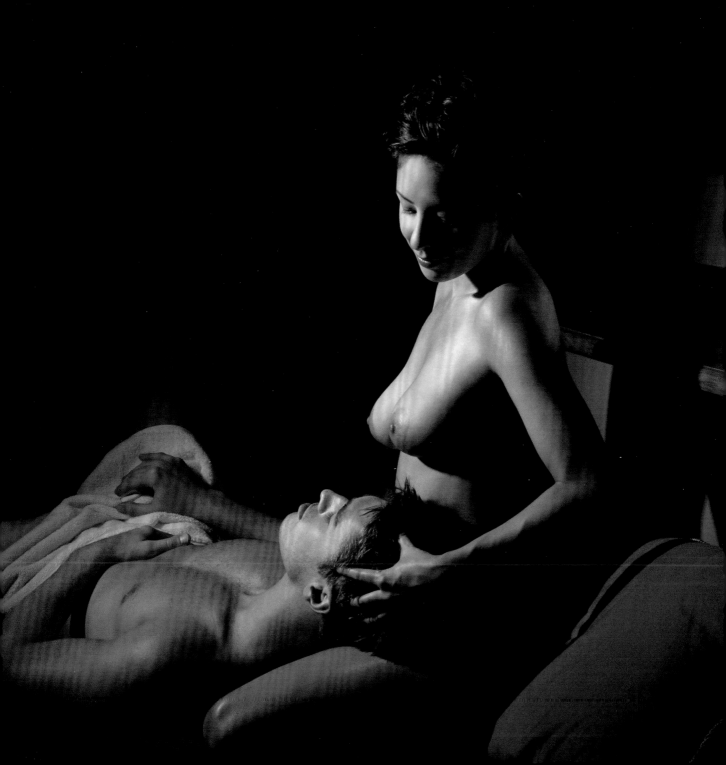

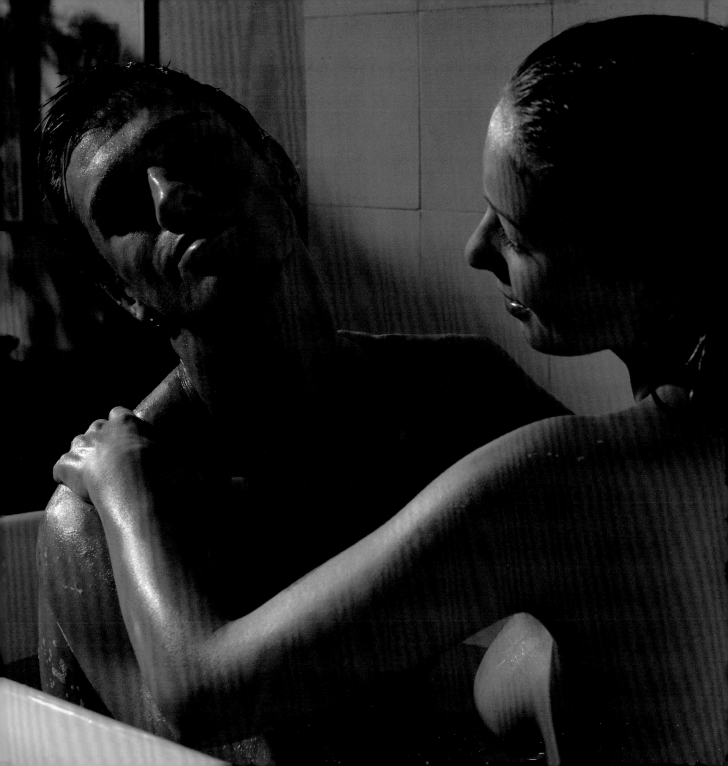

Taste

Although you may not be accustomed to eating while you bathe, food and drink *do* have a place in the bathroom. From a purely practical standpoint, hot water is dehydrating, so a tall glass of cold water is a necessity. But since a sensual bath is focused on pleasing all five senses, give your sense of taste equal consideration as sight, smell, hearing, and touch.

Don't expect your lover to feed you a four-course meal in the tub; nor should you eat a plate of greasy chicken while enjoying a solo sensual bath. The object is not to gratify your hunger, but to stimulate your sense of taste. Keep the fare light and the portions small, focusing on flavor and practical, bite-sized portions.

Create your own taste sensation or try one of these combinations:

- Ice-cold water with slices of lemon, frozen grapes
- Sweet white wine, such as Sauvignon Blanc or Gewürztraminer, and squares of dark chocolate
- Cold champagne, ripe strawberries
- Iced tea with fresh mint, sliced green apple, sharp Cheddar cheese
- Red wine, fresh figs, roasted almonds

Part of the appeal of fine food is visual presentation. To make your experience even more memorable, arrange a tray with sparkling crystal, fine china and a cloth napkin. Add a rose in a bud vase, and place the tray on a stool within easy reach of the tub. Take turns feeding one another tidbits of food. Focus on the taste and texture of the food and drink, allowing the flavor to blend with the other sensual elements in the room.

AFTER YOU'VE ASSEMBLED all that's necessary to prepare your physical and sensual environments, you're ready to enjoy the pleasures of your hard work and draw yourself a bath.

Spice It Up

LIKE WATER FOR CHOCOLATE

If you and your lover are so inclined, the bath is a fabulous place to play with food. Pour warm chocolate sauce over her body and lick her clean; eat whipped cream off his chest and belly. Don't be afraid to get messy—cleanup will be a breeze.

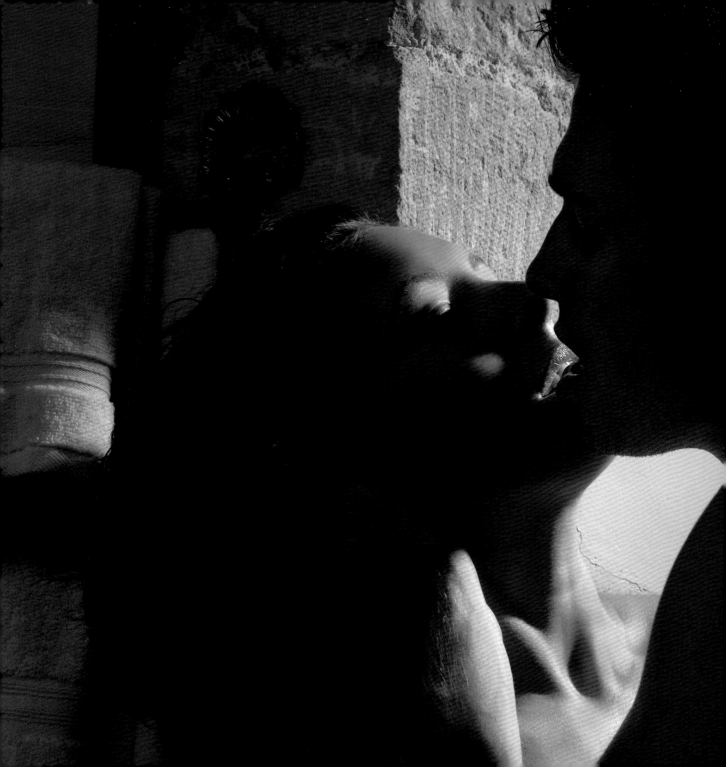

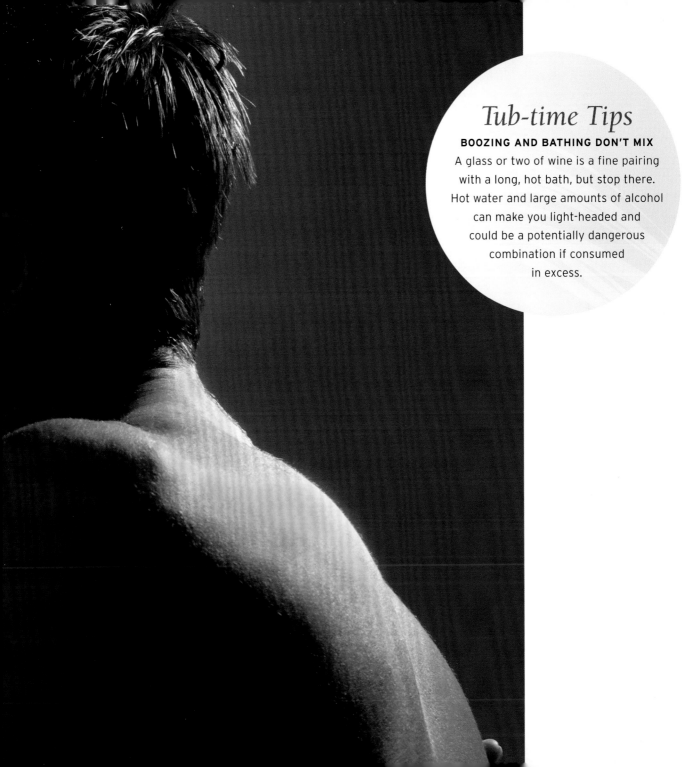

Tub-time Tips

BOOZING AND BATHING DON'T MIX

A glass or two of wine is a fine pairing
with a long, hot bath, but stop there.
Hot water and large amounts of alcohol
can make you light-headed and
could be a potentially dangerous
combination if consumed
in excess.

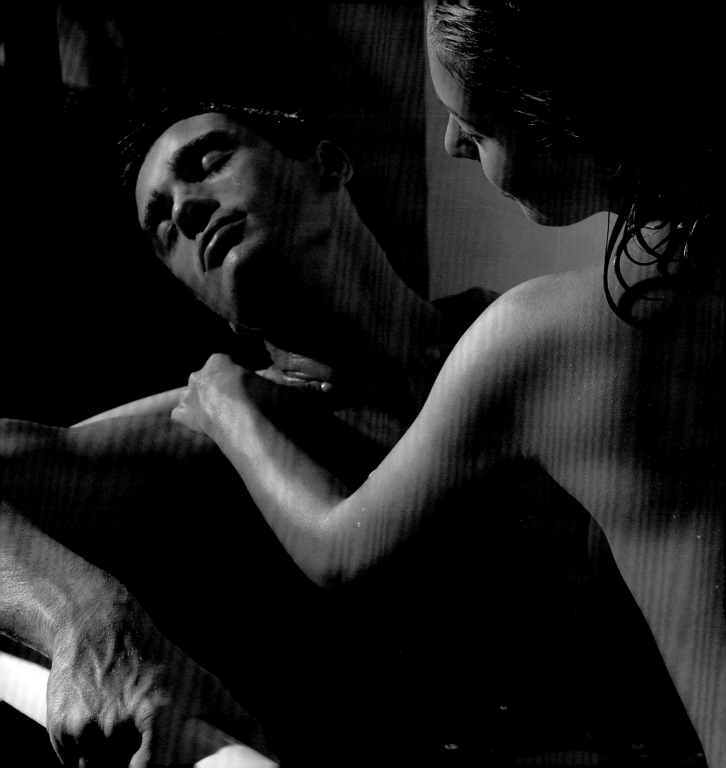

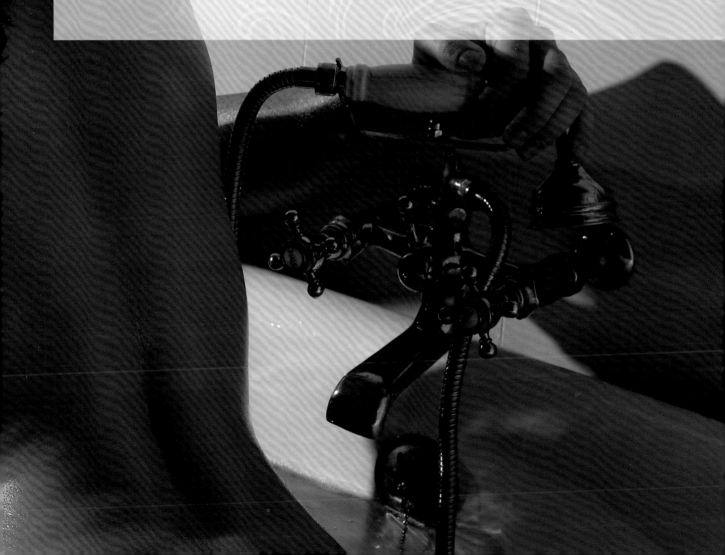

Chapter 4

Pampering Your Body

INDULGING YOUR SENSUAL SELF

CARING FOR YOUR BODY is the ultimate form of self-love. As you exfoliate your skin, moisturize your hair and rub thick cream into your hands and feet, you reconnect with your most basic self, the pleasure-loving hedonist that delights in feeling clean and pampered. Instead of limiting your enjoyment of these homemade body treatments to solo baths, introduce your partner to pampering by integrating a skin, hair, hand, or foot treatment into your sensual bath.

THROUGHOUT HISTORY women have known the pleasures of indulging themselves with beauty treatments, while men have just begun to catch up. There's no reason why people of either sex can't enjoy the benefits of an invigorating body scrub or a deep-cleaning hair mask—especially when administered by a loving partner. By caring for each other's bodies, we satisfy our basic human need to nurture, which in turn makes us feel good. Have fun with each other: Giggle at how you look with a clay mask on your face or write your initials on his back in exfoliating scrub. If the mood turns romantic, indulge in that, too—as soon as you rinse off!

Store-bought products are fine for everyday bathing, but when you're indulging in a sensual bath, alone or with a partner, you deserve the luxury of some homemade pampering. Inexpensive and easy to assemble, the scrubs, masks, and treatments in this chapter use natural, organic ingredients commonly found in grocery and health-food stores nationwide. If you're worried about your lack of culinary skills, then relax; you won't be doing anything more than measuring and mixing ingredients.

Skin Treatments

When it comes to caring for your skin, you need to do three things: cleanse, exfoliate, and moisturize. Cleansing is easy—everyone knows what soap and water are for. Moisturizing is also a no-brainer; women can choose from a thousand different hydrating products and even rugged guys appreciate the need for a little lotion.

Exfoliating is a little trickier, but anyone who's ever had an itch in that unreachable spot in the middle of his back will appreciate the need for getting rid of dead skin. By sloughing off old, dull cells, we make way for healthy, new skin. Whether you choose to see that metaphorically or not is up to you, but in reality, scrubbing each other feels good, so why not go for it?

Body Scrubs

In past times, we concocted homemade skin treatments from oatmeal, honey, and avocado. Nowadays, we know better: salt or sugar body scrubs are most beneficial to the skin. Granules of sugar or salt exfoliate the skin, while oils moisturize, so you get an added bonus every time you use one of these scrubs. Plus, there's no unpleasant chafing, as with oatmeal or apricot scrubs, so these scrubs are good for all skin types, even sensitive skin.

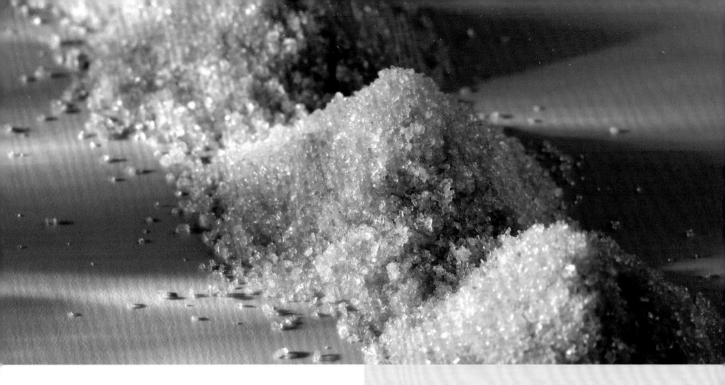

You can purchase these tingly, moisturizing balms just about anywhere—the mall, the grocery store, the Internet—but since they are so easy and inexpensive to make, impress your partner by whipping up your own batch and surprising him or her in the shower. None of these recipes takes longer than a few minutes to combine, and you don't need any expertise.

Using these scrubs is the fun part. As you rub the scrub into your skin, the sugar or salt will slowly melt, sloughing away dead skin cells and leaving behind deeply moisturized skin. Use gentle, circular motions to work the scrub into your skin until the sugar or salt completely dissolves, and then rinse with warm water. At first, it may feel like you still have oily residue on your skin, but that's just a trick of the water. When you're dry, your skin will feel soft, smooth, and clean.

Spice It Up

JUST ADD WATER

A delightful side effect of using a salt or sugar scrub is the chemistry that happens when you get wet again. Try it with a partner: scrub each other, rinse, dry off, and then drizzle water over strategic parts of your anatomy— breasts, thighs, bellies. The water will revive the oil moisturizing your skin; slide up against your partner for a special kind of slipperiness.

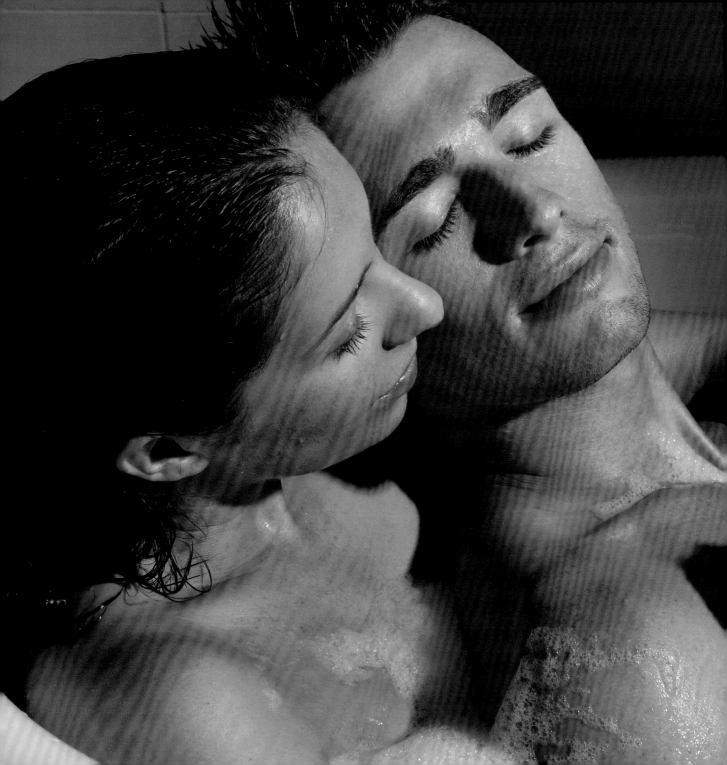

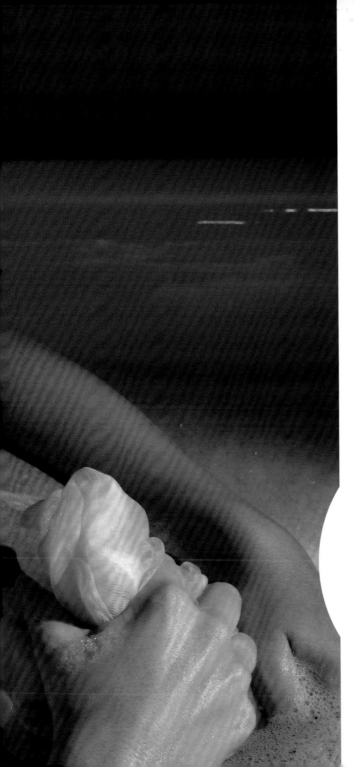

Salt Scrubs

If you've never used a salt scrub before, you might find the experience a little peculiar at first. The texture of the scrub itself is unusual, neither rough nor smooth, but a hybrid that somehow exfoliates and moisturizes your skin at the same time. When you rub it into your skin, it's rough at first, but then it melts away, leaving what seems to be a greasy residue. Dry your skin, however, and you'll find it's anything but oily—it will feel smooth, clean, and incredibly soft.

Don't use salt scrubs on anything delicate, like your eyes, face, or genitals, although all other body parts are fine. Some people like to rinse off the scrub right away, and others prefer to let the scrub set for a few minutes before rinsing it off. It's up to you, but just avoid using a salt scrub more than once a week.

Tub-time Tips

PATCH TEST

Before applying any kind of skin product, make sure you aren't allergic to any of the ingredients. Dab a bit of the mixture you're using onto your wrist. If after several minutes your skin doesn't burn or itch unpleasantly, it should be safe to use.

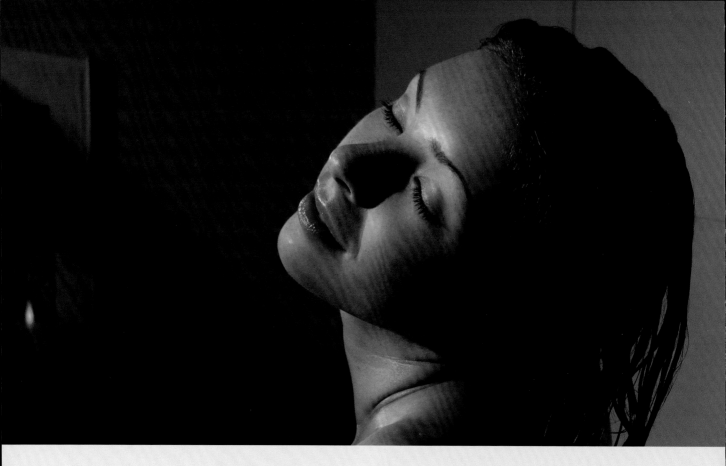

When I was a teenager I consistently used apricot body scrub on my face, neck, shoulders, back, and chest—anywhere I could reach. A few years ago, I rediscovered this sensual pleasure in a brown-sugar body scrub my niece gave me for my birthday. The rough, buttery texture feels even better than the scrub I remembered, and my skin feels a thousand times softer when I'm done.

—*Michelle, 38*

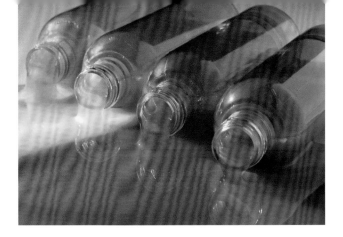

The following recipes are different salt scrubs that you might try to cleanse and moisturize your skin, leaving you feeling smooth and luscious for some sensual play after your sensual bath.

- **Relaxing Scrub**

  The soothing fragrance of lavender makes this scrub a perfect choice for relaxing solo baths or romantic evenings with a partner. If you find the scrub too thick in texture, add up to a tablespoon of olive oil until you reach a consistency you like. This recipe makes enough for one person, but it is very easily doubled (or tripled!).

  INGREDIENTS
  2 cups (600 g) Epsom salt
  ¼ cup (60 ml) Vaseline
  10 drops lavender essential oil

  Pour Epsom salt into a small bowl. Add Vaseline and blend with a spoon until evenly mixed. Add essential oils and blend until smooth. Use immediately.

- **Ginger-Peppermint Body Scrub**

  This refreshing and invigorating scrub will awaken your senses and leave your skin smooth, soft, and moisturized. Although just about everyone can enjoy this scrub, it is especially good to use with a partner, so this recipe yields enough for two people to enjoy. If you're bathing alone, halve the recipe. You can also double the recipe, but it doesn't keep, so don't make more than you'll use in one bath.

  INGREDIENTS
  ½ cup (150 g) sea salt
  ½ cup (80 g) cornmeal
  ⅔ cup (160 ml) olive oil
  1 tablespoon (10 g) fresh ginger,
      peeled and finely minced
  10 drops peppermint essential oil

  In a small bowl, mix the salt and cornmeal. Pour olive oil into a medium bowl and heat until warm. Add essential oils. A little at a time, add the dry ingredients, mixing well until blended. Add ginger and blend until the scrub is completely smooth and even in texture. Use immediately.

- **Manly Man Mix**

  If your man starts complaining that everything smells like flowers, treat him to a big batch of this very manly scrub. The bay leaves and cedarwood give a deep, earthy base to the eucalyptus oil, which refreshes and invigorates.

INGREDIENTS

¼ cup (75 g) sea salt
¼ cup (75 g) Epsom salt
4 dried bay leaves, pulverized
½ cup (120 ml) olive oil
5 drops eucalyptus essential oil
5 drops cedarwood essential oil

In a medium bowl, mix together the sea salt, Epsom salt and bay leaves. Slowly add the oil, stirring until evenly blended. Add essential oil and mix thoroughly. Use immediately. (Recipe yields enough scrub to thoroughly scrub one large, manly man.)

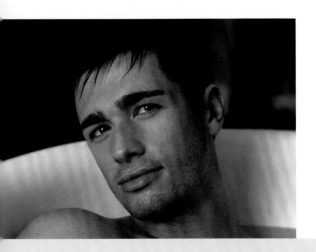

My lover's hands *are warm and gentle as they rub thick, luscious, lavender-scented scrub onto my wet body. At first, the salt feels coarse against my breasts and arms, but as it dissolves against my skin, the tingling feels wonderful, the slight scraping delicious, especially over my back and buttocks. After the granules have melted away, there is only my damp, silky skin and my lover's hands on my body.*

—Laura, 32

Sugar Scrubs

Sugar is an excellent exfoliant for two reasons: chemistry and texture. Sugar cane supplies the world with a multitude of useful products, only one of which is the sinful ingredient that makes cookies so delicious. Another product is glycolic acid, one of the few alpha hydroxy acids found in nature. A key ingredient to most skincare products designed to reduce wrinkles and help problem skin, alpha hydroxy acids exfoliate the skin, removing dead cells and other impurities.

Regular granulated sugar possesses two exfoliating properties: glycolic acid and a rough texture. It's also one of the cheapest beauty-treatment ingredients you'll find! You won't need high-quality sugar for any of these scrubs—pick up a few pounds at any grocery store. Because sugar scrubs are the essence of sweetness, you may prefer to use sweet almond oil instead of olive oil. Experiment with both and use what works for you.

Use sugar scrubs the same way you'd use salt scrubs: Gently rub a small handful into your skin until the rough texture disappears, leaving behind soft, moisturized skin. You might feel a little oily at first, but once you dry yourself off, your skin will feel clean and silky. You will stay slippery while wet, so be careful walking around on tile, at least until you're dry. Also, these scrubs don't keep very well, so try not to make more than you can use at one time. If you must, you can refrigerate leftovers for up to 10 days.

The following recipes are for various sugar scrubs that you can make at home, which will your leave your skin feeling extra soft!

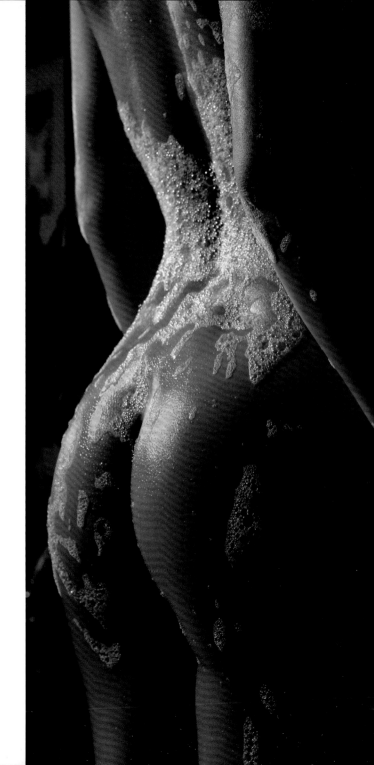

- **Simple Sugar Scrub**

  Not only is this scrub easy to make, but it's also simple to adapt to your mood. Choose lavender and rosemary essential oils for a soothing scrub; jasmine, patchouli, or ylang-ylang for romance; peppermint to invigorate; or a custom blend you create. For an unscented version, skip the essential oils altogether. This recipe yields enough for one thorough scrubbing. If you want to make a bigger batch, just keep the ingredients in proportion and make as much as you need.

  INGREDIENTS
  ½ cup (100 g) granulated sugar
  ½ cup (120 ml) olive oil
  1 tablespoon (15 ml) aloe vera gel
  5 drops essential oil

  In a small bowl, blend the sugar and olive oil. Add the aloe vera gel and essential oil and mix until smooth. Use immediately and refrigerate unused portion.

Keeping It Simple

One of the main principles behind homemade beauty treatments is keeping it simple. Pricier oils, produce, and supplies aren't going to provide greater benefits to your skin or hair, so don't waste your time or money hunting down unusual, expensive versions of ingredients you can buy for next to nothing. Olive oil makes the best base for salt and sugar scrubs, but there's no need to splurge on imported extra-virgin oil. You can also use almond oil, especially if you like the sweet scent, but it's a bit pricier and not as easy to find. Avoid baby oil; it's too thin to work well with sugar or salt scrubs.

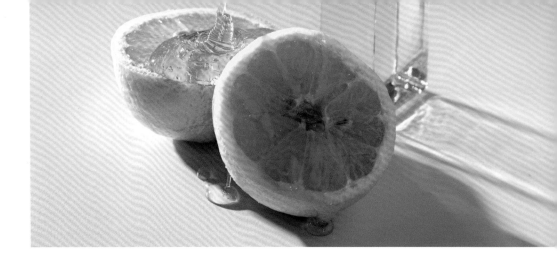

- **Soothing Lemon Scrub**

  The perfect choice when you want to feel extra-pampered, this scrub is as soothing as a cup of lemon tea with honey. The sweet, tart fragrance will please your senses; if you especially like lemony scents, add more lemon essential oil or lemon juice. If you find the mixture too dilute, add another ¼ to ½ cup (50 to 100 g) of sugar. Yields enough scrub for two people.

  INGREDIENTS

  2 cups (400 g) sugar
  ½ cup (120 ml) sweet almond oil
  1 tablespoon (15 ml) lemon juice
  ¼ cup (60 ml) honey
  5 drops lemon essential oil

  In a medium bowl, combine the sugar and sweet almond oil, blending until the mixture is consistent in texture. Add the lemon juice and honey, and mix well. Add essential oil and blend thoroughly. Use immediately and refrigerate unused portion.

- **Sweet and Silky Scrub**

  Powdered milk gives this sugar scrub a smooth, luxuriant feel; the sweet fragrance will appeal to your sense of romance. Don't use real milk or your scrub will be soupy!

  INGREDIENTS

  1 cup (200 g) granulated or brown sugar
  2 cups (230 g) powdered milk
  1 cup (240 ml) olive oil
  10 drops jasmine or rose essential oil

  In a medium bowl, mix together the sugar and powdered milk. Slowly add the olive oil, stirring continuously. The mixture should be gritty and coarse; add more or less oil until you reach a consistency you like. Add essential oils and blend well.

Facial Treatments

The skin on your face is more sensitive than the skin on your arms and legs, so treat it accordingly with a mask specific to your skin type. If you find that a mask irritates your skin, don't use it again; however, keep in mind that exfoliating masks sometimes cause initial redness or dryness that goes away in a day or two. Limit facials to once a week, and follow a few basic guidelines:

- Use bottled or distilled water in all facial treatments. Hard water can be high in skin-irritant minerals. If you're confined only to tap water, boil it first to cleanse it of impurities.

- Before you apply a mask, spend a few minutes enjoying the pore-opening steam in your shower or bath, and then cleanse your face and neck thoroughly with warm water.

- When applying a mask, start in the middle of your forehead, moving in circular motions down your temples and across your cheeks, covering your nose, chin, upper lip, and throat. Leave a clean space around your eyes and mouth, where the skin is extra sensitive.

- Don't leave a mask on longer than the recommended time or you risk a breakout or irritated skin. Rinse with warm water and pat dry.

- When your bath is over, wipe your skin with a toning liquid; witch hazel is a safe, inexpensive alternative to pricy store astringents. Follow up with a rich moisturizer.

- Facials can cause initial redness or breakouts, especially if you are clearing your skin of a lot of impurities. Don't experiment with a new facial the day before your wedding, family portrait sitting, or big presentation at work.

Toner Facial

The essential step between cleansing and moisturizing, skin toner tightens your pores and preps your skin for hydration. Saturate a couple of cotton balls or squares and stroke the toner over your face, throat, neck, chest, and shoulders.

The following recipe for rosewater skin toner will not only cleanse, but also hydrate your skin, giving you an all-around brighter and softer appearance.

- **Rosewater Skin Tonic**
  A gentle, fragrant astringent, this toner will close your pores and condition your skin. If you find the lemon too acidic, reduce it by 10 percent until you find a balance that works for your skin. This recipe yields about 18 ounces (540 ml) of toner.

  INGREDIENTS
  1 cup (240 ml) witch hazel
  1 cup (240 ml) rose water
  ¼ cup (60 ml) fresh lemon juice, strained

  In a clean bottle, combine all ingredients. Shake gently to blend. Store in a cool dark place for up to two weeks.

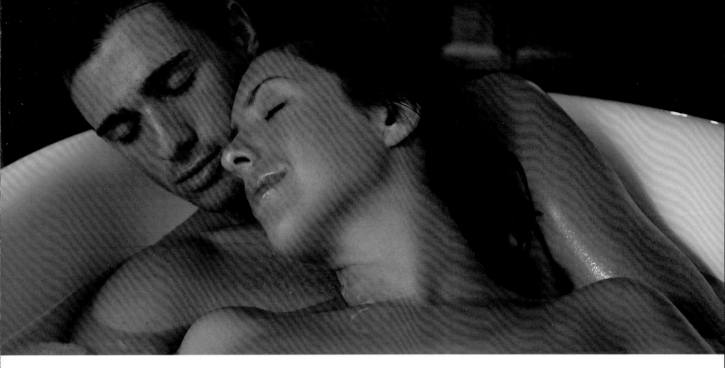

Facials for Oily/Combination Skin

These following facial treatments cleanse your pores
and eliminate impurities that could result in breakouts.

- **"Breakfast" Facial**

    In this skin treatment, the oatmeal exfoliates and
    moisturizes, and the egg purifies and tightens
    your pores. Since it's not the most visually
    appealing of facial treatments, you might want
    to save this one for the solo bath, since it might
    not be considered a sexy addition to your
    sensual bath!

INGREDIENTS
¼ cup (22 g) dry rolled oats
1 large egg, separated

In a small bowl, break open and separate the egg,
discarding the yolk. Add the oatmeal to the egg
white and mix into a thick paste. Apply the
mixture to your face and neck, letting it sit for up
to 15 minutes. Rinse thoroughly with warm water
and pat your skin dry.

Sink-top Sauna

If you don't have time to steam open your pores with a bath or shower, try this quickie countertop version. Boil three cups of water and pour it into a heat-safe bowl. Add five drops of one or more essential oils recommended for your skin type:

- Normal/Combination Skin: Orange, bergamot, lavender
- Oily Skin: Lemon, peppermint, rosemary, eucalyptus
- Dry Skin: Rose, ylang-ylang, chamomile, jasmine

With your face about nine inches from the fragrant water, cover your head with a clean bath towel. Let the steam work for about three minutes, and then rinse your face with clean warm water.

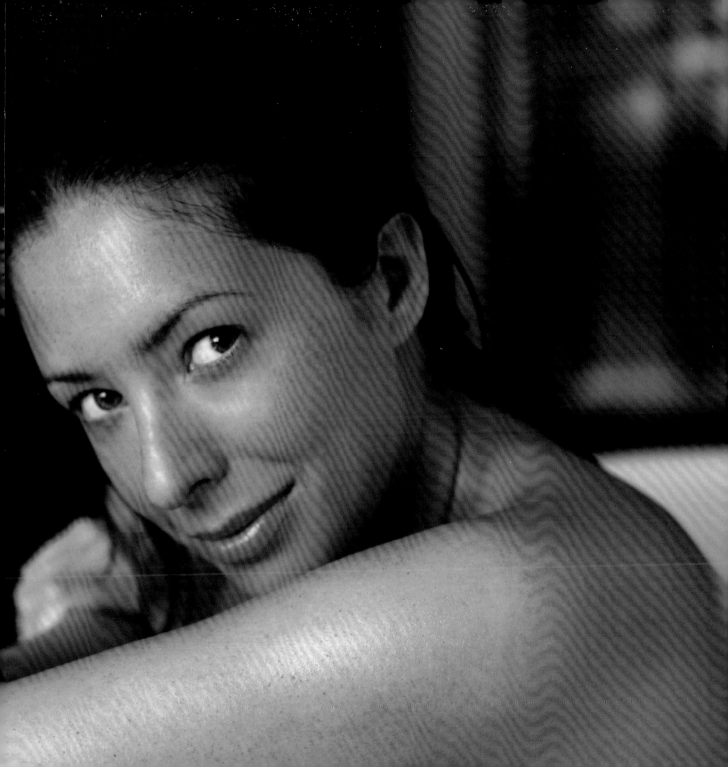

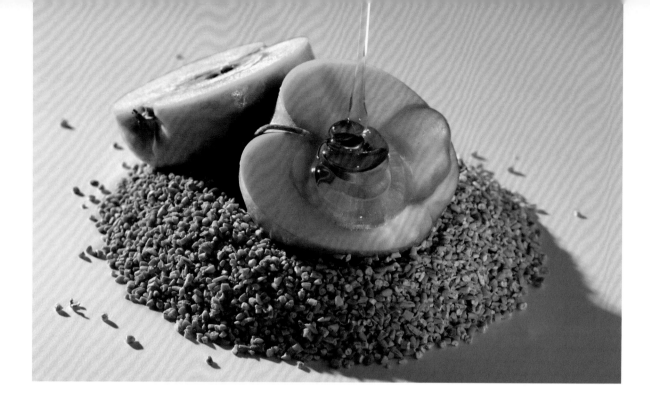

- **Apple Pie Facial**

  The acidic mixture of apple puree and lemon juice invigorates oily skin, the oatmeal exfoliates, and the honey keeps the whole mess together. Another not-so-sexy facial treatment, this one is ridiculous-looking enough to be fun for playful couples, so this recipe yields enough mask for two.

  INGREDIENTS
  1 large apple, peeled, cored, and finely grated
      or pureed in a food processor
  1 tablespoon (15 ml) fresh lemon juice, strained
  ½ cup (120 ml) honey
  ¼ cup (22 g) rolled oats

  In a small bowl, combine the apple and lemon juice. Add the honey and stir well. Mix in the oatmeal and stir until thoroughly blended. To adjust the consistency, add more or less honey. Apply to your face and throat and let sit for up to 10 minutes. Rinse thoroughly with cool water.

- **Basic Clay Mask**

  Available at natural food stores, fuller's earth is a clay compound that removes impurities from skin. If you have sensitive skin, substitute French green clay, also available at any health-food store. Adapt this basic recipe with your own favorite essential oils, or use the mask unscented.

INGREDIENTS

1 tablespoon (15 ml) fuller's earth or
    French green clay

2 tablespoons (30 ml) water

1 teaspoon (5 ml) honey

3 drops lavender essential oil (optional)

Measure clay into a small dish and carefully add water. Stir until smoothly blended. Add honey and mix well. If the mixture seems too runny, add more honey; smooth out a rich mask with water. When the mixture reaches your desired consistency, blend in the essential oil. Apply evenly over your face and throat and allow the mask to set for up to 15 minutes. Rinse your skin thoroughly with warm water. To remove all traces of the clay, follow up with a toner.

Tea Tree Oil

Distilled from the leaves of Australia native *Melaleuca alternifolia*, tea tree oil is a distinctive-smelling essential oil with a variety of useful properties. Added to bath oil or beauty treatments, tea tree oil soothes skin irritated by insect bites and acne. Applied directly to blemishes, it's an excellent spot-treatment for pimples. It might not sound all that sexy, but its bracing aroma and soothing properties make tea tree oil a worthy addition to any sensual apothecary.

Facials for Dry and Sensitive Skin

These all-natural treatments hydrate dry skin and calm irritated or troubled skin. If you have sensitive skin, test each mixture on the inside of your wrist before applying the mask to your face.

The following recipes for moisturizing masks can be used on the face, neck, throat, chest, back, and shoulders.

- **Moisturizing Oatmeal Mask**
  Although oatmeal is often used as an exfoliant, it's also an excellent natural moisturizer, especially when combined with creamy milk and super-hydrating honey.

  INGREDIENTS
  ½ cup (45 g) dry rolled oats
  2 tablespoons (30 ml) milk
  1 tablespoon (15 ml) honey

  In a small bowl, combine the oats and milk, thickening the mixture with honey until it reaches the consistency of a thick paste. Apply to your face and neck and leave for up to ten minutes. Rinse with cool water and pat your skin dry gently.

- **Egg Cream Hydrating Mask**
  This mask smells pleasant and resembles a light glaze, making it a great pick for facials *à deux*. Although you shouldn't eat the mask (raw egg can carry salmonella), it's safe to use on your face, neck, and torso. This recipe makes enough for two to enjoy.

  INGREDIENTS
  2 egg yolks
  3 tablespoons (45 ml) olive oil
  1 teaspoon (5 ml) fresh lemon juice, strained

  In a small bowl, pierce egg yolks and scramble slightly. Slowly add the oil, mixing consistently until mixture is emulsified. Add lemon juice and blend thoroughly. Apply to skin in a thin, even layer. After 10 minutes, rinse with warm water.

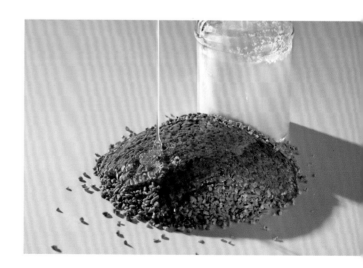

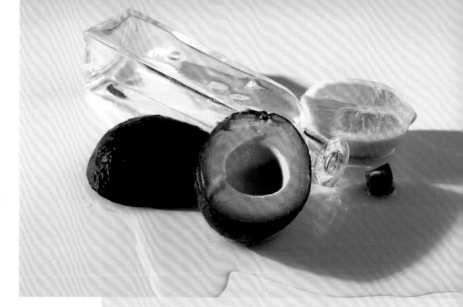

- **Avocado Face Butter**

  While this might not be the sexiest mask, this green, gooey butter nonetheless smells delicious and works wonders for dry or sun-damaged skin. This recipe yields one facial mask. If you want to share this experience with your partner, feel free to double the recipe.

INGREDIENTS

1 ripe avocado, peeled, seeded and
    mashed
1 tablespoon (15 ml) olive oil
3 drops rosemary essential oil
1 teaspoon (5 ml) lemon juice (optional)

In a bowl, blend avocado and olive oil until smooth. If you'd like a more diluted facial, thin the mixture with lemon juice. Add rosemary essential oil and blend thoroughly. Apply to face and throat, being sure to avoid your eyes and mouth. Leave on for up to 20 minutes and then rinse thoroughly with cool water.

Exfoliating Skin Treatments

Exfoliating masks help rid your skin of dead cells and other pore-clogging impurities, leaving your face smooth, clean, and soft. Like exfoliating body scrubs, exfoliating masks are fun to use alone or with a partner.

Spice It Up

THERAPEUTIC MUD WRESTLING?

Masks aren't just for faces! You and your partner can turn up the heat by turning your facial into a skin treatment for your necks, backs, shoulders, and chests. Smooth the treatment evenly over one another's skin, and while you're waiting for it to work, sit back in the tub together and relax. When it's time to rinse off the mask, you and your partner can have some dirty fun making sure every inch of skin is squeaky clean.

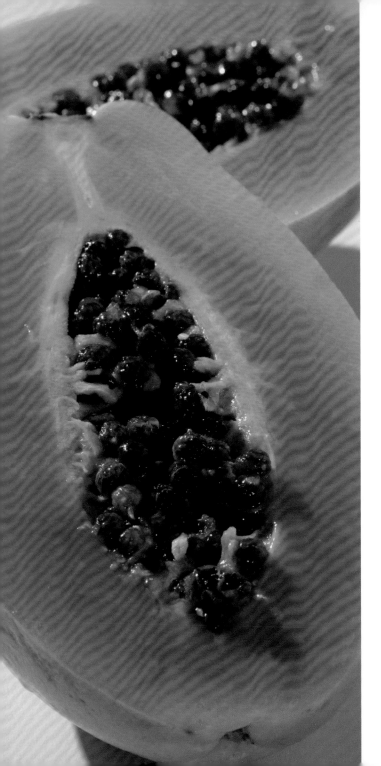

The following exfoliating mask recipes not only will leave your skin glowing, but the textures are interesting, and the treatments smell delicious.

- **Papaya Pumpkin Enzymatic Exfoliant**
  This beauty treatment is worthy of its grandiose title and somewhat complicated preparation. Papaya and pumpkin both contain enzymes that are among the most powerful found in nature. Combining both in one mask is sheer brilliance. This recipe yields more than enough for two.

INGREDIENTS
1 egg white
1 teaspoon (5 ml) honey
½ ripe papaya, skinned, seeded, and mashed
1 cup (240 ml) canned pumpkin puree

Using a handheld mixer, whip egg white until frothy; blend in honey. Gradually add the papaya and pumpkin, blending continuously until all ingredients are evenly mixed. Beat on high for one minute. Fold mixture into an airtight container and refrigerate for up to two weeks.

    To use the mask, apply evenly over your face, neck, and throat, being careful to avoid the sensitive skin around your eyes. After five minutes, rinse thoroughly with cool water.

- **Boozy Sloughing Mask**

  If the man in your life balks at "girly" skin treatments, surprise him with this stout mixture. If he still complains, tell him to look into the science behind this recipe: the beer, barley, and honey have a chemical reaction with the lime juice, the product of which sloughs away dead, dry skin. If nothing else, he'll enjoy the heady aroma! Barley powder is widely available at natural food stores.

  INGREDIENTS

  2 tablespoons (30 ml) barley powder

  1 tablespoon (15 ml) honey

  1 tablespoon (15 ml) warm beer

  1 tablespoon (15 ml) lime juice

  In a bowl, mix together the barley powder and honey. Add the beer and blend well. Squeeze in the lime juice and mix thoroughly. Apply mixture to his face and neck. After 10 minutes, rinse with warm water.

HAIR TREATMENTS

LIKE SKIN, hair is a self-renewing resource, provided you give it a little extra TLC every once in a while. People with short hair might not see the point of all that pampering, but hair of any length will benefit from these treatments.

Shinier Hair

Although old wives would have you believe that your kitchen is crammed with products that will make your hair look healthier, the truth is that everyone's hair dulls naturally over time. Add back some shine with one of these color-appropriate rinses:

- **Blondes:** Lemon juice
- **Redheads:** Cider vinegar
- **Brunettes:** Coffee grounds

  Preparation is the same for all three rinses: Add one tablespoon of your chosen material to a quart of room-temperature distilled or bottled water. After you've shampooed, conditioned, and rinsed clean your hair, slowly pour the shine rinse over your head. Gently shake away the excess and wrap your hair in a towel. You'll see shinier locks when your hair dries. The effect isn't permanent, so repeat as often as once a week for more luxurious locks.

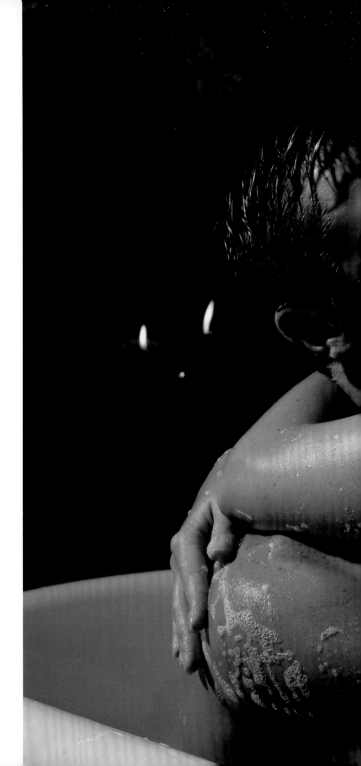

Color-enhancing Herbal Rinses

Similar to shine-enhancing rinses, color-enhancing rinses leverage nature's floral bounty to temporarily boost the predominant color in your hair. If chemistry scares you, don't panic. These rinses are not so much hard science as they are culinary wizardry.

All you'll need is a large saucepan, a 12-inch (30-cm) square of doubled cheesecloth (available at any grocery store), a piece of string, a wooden spoon, the ability to boil water, and one of the following color-specific herbs, available at natural food stores or via the Internet.

- **Blonde:** dried whole chamomile flowers
- **Brunette:** crushed fresh rosemary sprigs
- **Redhead:** crumpled fresh hibiscus petals (if your retailer doesn't have these, your neighbor's shrub might lend a few—ask first!)
- **Silver Tones:** dried hollyhock flowers

Over high heat, boil a quart of water. While you're waiting, spread the cheesecloth open in a double layer and place your selected herb in the middle. Use a piece of string to tie the herb into a secure bundle. Add the package to the boiling water, using a wooden spoon to push the bundle to the bottom of the pot, anchoring it in place with the spoon. Turn off the heat and let the concoction steep and cool for about 20 minutes. Use the spoon to fish out the bundle.

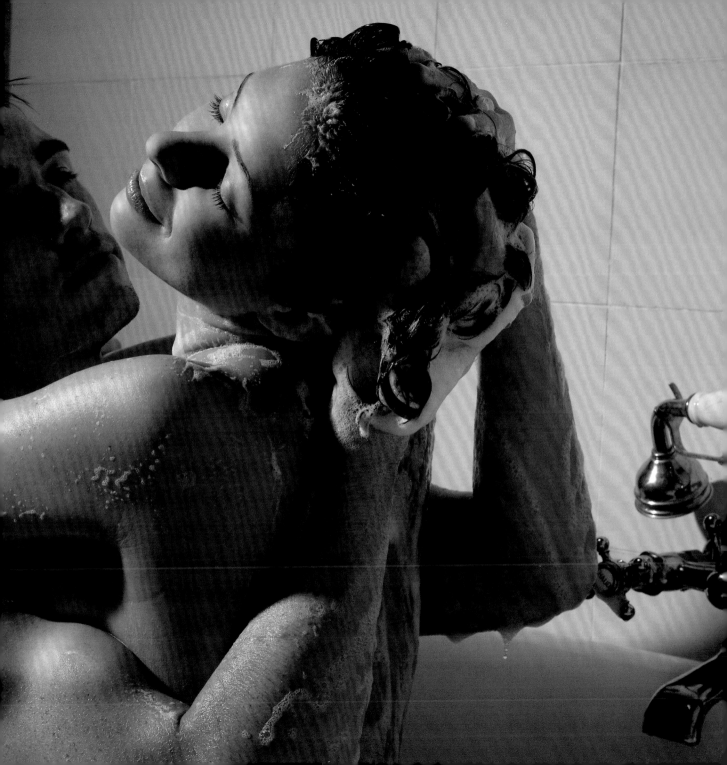

After you shampoo, condition, and rinse your hair, slowly pour the herbal brew over your clean locks. Allow the mixture to drip through for a few minutes while you comb out your wet hair. Rinse with cool water and towel dry.

Like the shine-boosting rinses, these color rinses are temporary. Repeat as frequently as twice a month to keep your hair vibrant.

Henna

Since ancient times, women around the world have used henna to add natural, temporary red tones to red, brown, and dark brunette hair. Native to Africa, Southeast Asia, and Australia, the henna plant is a small flowering shrub that produces a red-orange substance that bonds easily with protein. Since much of our epidermal layer—our hair, skin, and nails—is comprised of proteins, henna is an effective dye well-suited to temporary body art and hair rinses. Today, henna paste is available at natural food, specialty, and ethnic stores nationwide and online.

To add glossy, temporary red tones to your natural or color-processed hair, prepare the paste according to the package instructions, working it through clean, wet hair. Use a wide-toothed comb to distribute the paste evenly from root to end, and then pin up your hair and cover it with a plastic shower cap or with plastic wrap. Let the paste sit for two to four hours, depending on the intensity of color you desire. Start with less time and work your way up to richer tones. Rinse your hair with cool water until the water runs clear—and then rinse it a few more times for good measure. Repeat as often as once a month.

Henna will not damage your hair, but until you know how the color of the dye interacts with your specific hair color, you'll want to proceed with caution so you don't wind up with tomato-red instead of bright auburn. Also, like commercial hair dyes, henna will discolor your skin, clothing, and linens, so always wear gloves when applying the rinse and take care to guard your skin and clothing against drips. Clean up any spills immediately.

Moisturizing Hair Masks

Most DIY hair treatments seem to function on the same mathematical equation: Food + Heat + Time = Soft Hair. No matter what your favorite hydrating food combinations, the process is the same:

- Apply "food" mixture to dry hair. Most of these hair masks are slippery and challenging to work with; you'll have an easier time working with dry hair. You'll wash out the treatment with shampoo, so don't worry about becoming a walking pantry.
- Wrap head in plasic wrap. If you have long hair, hold your hair in a ponytail at the back of your head and wind a 24- to 36-inch piece of plastic wrap around it, beginning at the base of the ponytail and spiraling down to the ends. Then wrap that bundle around your head with another piece of plastic wrap. Cover with a pretty shower cap or a plush towel wrapped turban-style.

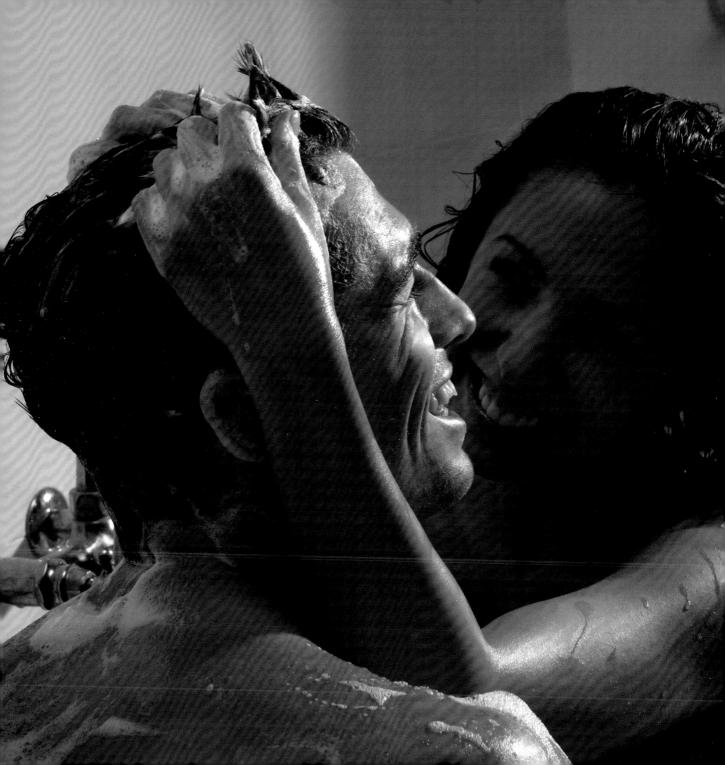

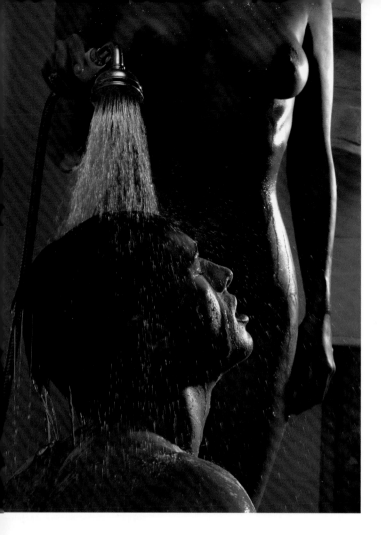

- Relax in a hot, steamy bath. While you're soaking, the heat will penetrate all those layers of plastic and activate the hydrating agent in the mask. If your hair is dry and damaged, keep the mask on for up to 30 minutes. If your scalp is oily, apply the product to the ends of your hair only and soak for 20 minutes.
- Shampoo, rinse, and repeat. And, if possible, repeat again. The one downside to intensive moisturizing hair masks is that they all seem to be uniformly difficult to get out of your hair. If your hair is especially thick, try a clarifying shampoo. Otherwise, baby shampoo should work to remove the ingredients from your soft, shiny hair.
- When your hair is completely clean and free of product, rinse with cold water. There's no need to condition your hair; just comb it through and enjoy your luscious locks.

YOU CAN SELECT your mask-making materials from one of the following kitchen staples discussed in the next section.

Mayonnaise

If you don't mind the smell, plain, old-fashioned mayo is possibly the most nourishing condiment you'll ever meet. It takes a while to work it through your hair—and it takes even longer to rinse it out—but the effort is worth it. Your hair will feel soft and shiny for days. It's best to save this treatment for solo baths.

Eggs

Although the yolk is the moisturizing portion of the egg, the whites help spread the hydration evenly over your whole head. Depending on how much hair you have, crack one or two—possibly three?—raw eggs into a bowl and mix lightly. Add the egg alone to your hair or, if you don't like runny masks, mix in a tablespoon of honey before applying.

Avocado

Rich in vitamin E, avocado is a delicious source of hydration for your hair. Peel, remove the pit, and mash a ripe avocado, applying it directly to your hair. Depending on your preference for aroma and texture, add a tablespoon of honey or lemon juice.

Olive Oil

Purists will enjoy keeping things simple with the most essential of all hair-care products: olive oil. Use as little or as much as you'd like, keeping in mind that the oil will not only hydrate your hair, but also condition your scalp. If you already tend toward the oily, skip this mask!

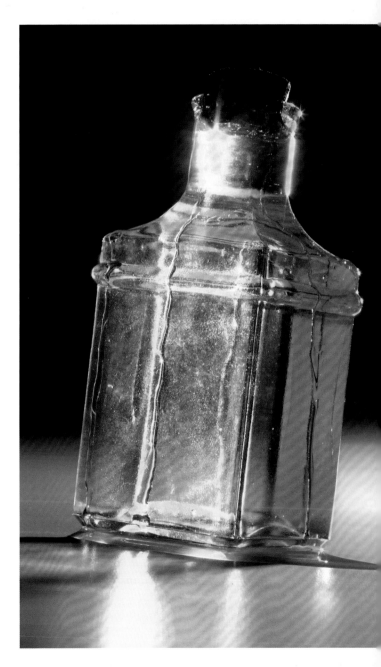

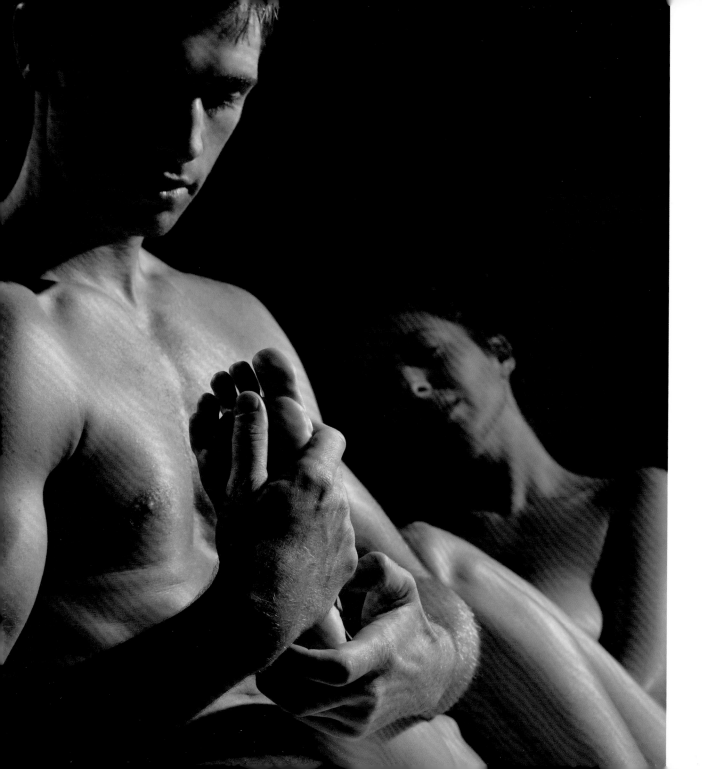

HAND AND FOOT TREATMENTS

AFTER ALL THE PAMPERING you're giving the rest of your body, don't neglect your hands and feet! Your extremities work hard all day; reward them with serious TLC.

These treatments are equally effective experienced alone or with your lover. Your objective should be relaxation, pleasure, and honoring your beautiful hands and feet. Some days, you might just want to engage in some solo therapy. However, every once in a while, you might feel like pampering your partner—or having him pamper *you*. On those occasions, make a production out of the event, using the techniques outlined in Chapter 3, "The Sensual Environment," to set the stage for romance.

Strawberry Hand and Foot Exfoliant

The acid in strawberries make them an excellent natural exfoliant, but the delicious taste and aphrodisiac properties of this summer favorite make it a particularly sensual pick. In a blender or food processor, puree a dozen ripe, stemmed strawberries. Add a quarter cup (60 ml) of olive oil and a tablespoon (15 ml) of sea salt, and blend until smooth. Massage the strawberry mixture into your hands and feet, and then rinse clean. Your fingers and toes will feel clean and invigorated.

Almond–Butter Overnight Cream

Why spend big bucks on fancy overnight creams for your hands and feet when you can make a better (and much more affordable!) product at home? All you need is sweet almond oil and regular unsalted butter. Blend together one tablespoon (15 ml) of oil for every cup of softened butter, using a hand mixer to smooth out any lumps. If you'd like, scent with a few drops of essential oil. Just before bed, slather your clean feet with the cream and slip on a pair of white cotton socks. Coat your hands with cream and put on white cotton gloves. Go to bed and dream about the soft hands and feet you'll have in the morning.

At-home Spa Paraffin Treatment

If you've ever had a fancy spa pedicure, you probably know all about the benefits of deep-conditioning rough hands and feet with melted paraffin wax.

For salon neophytes, this seemingly strange procedure truly appeals to the senses. Initially, the hot wax tingles with heat, but then it cools incredibly fast, forming a shell around your hands and feet, a process somewhat similar to ordering a chocolate-covered soft-serve ice cream cone at your local ice cream store—except, of course, for the fact that your appendages are covered with hot wax, not delicious fudge. And although you can technically eat paraffin, it's much more fun to break free of it. Afterward, your hands and feet will feel incredibly soft and smooth.

Hot Wax Hand and Foot Treatment

Once strictly the purview of pricey spas, paraffin treatments are now easy to do at home. Look for scented or unscented paraffin bars at grocery, craft, specialty, hardware, or bath-supply stores, or shop around online. This recipe makes enough for two sets of hands and feet.

INGREDIENTS AND SUPPLIES

Four 1-pound (450 g) bars of paraffin wax

Heat-safe container big enough for dipping

Thick moisturizing lotion

Plastic wrap

Essential oils (optional)

Following the package directions, melt the paraffin wax. Although you can use the stovetop method, the microwave is much faster, safer, and easier to clean up. Use a heat-safe container large enough to accommodate a hand or foot; add a few drops of your favorite essential oil if you'd like.

Carefully place the container of wax on the floor or on a low stool. Rub a thick layer of moisturizing lotion over one foot, and then dip your foot into the hot wax, removing it quickly. Wait a few seconds for the paraffin to harden slightly, and then dip your foot again. Repeat once more, so that you have three layers of wax evenly coating your foot from the ankle down.

Cover your waxy foot with the plastic wrap, making sure to cover every bit of wax, forming a tight seal. Repeat with your other foot, and then with each hand. Rest for about 15 minutes, letting the heat penetrate your skin. Remove the plastic wrap and peel away the now-cold paraffin. Your hands and feet will feel incredibly soft and smooth.

Spice It Up

SEXY WAX APPEAL!

The combination of sensations you'll experience with this wax treatment make it the perfect choice for partner play. The intense heat will titillate, and you'll have a good time playing with the wax. But before you even think about it, banish any idea of using the wax on anything other than hands or feet. This is a PG-rated beauty treatment! Of course, what you do *after* the treatment is up to you . . .

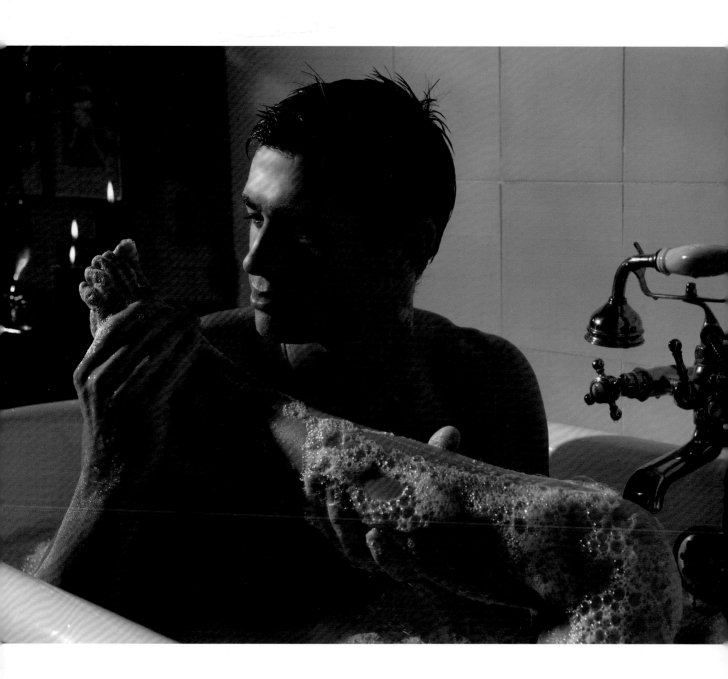

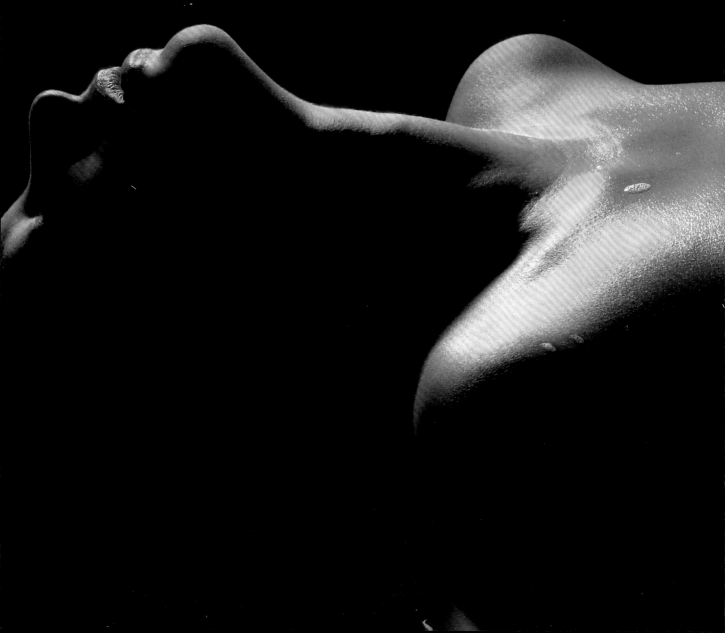

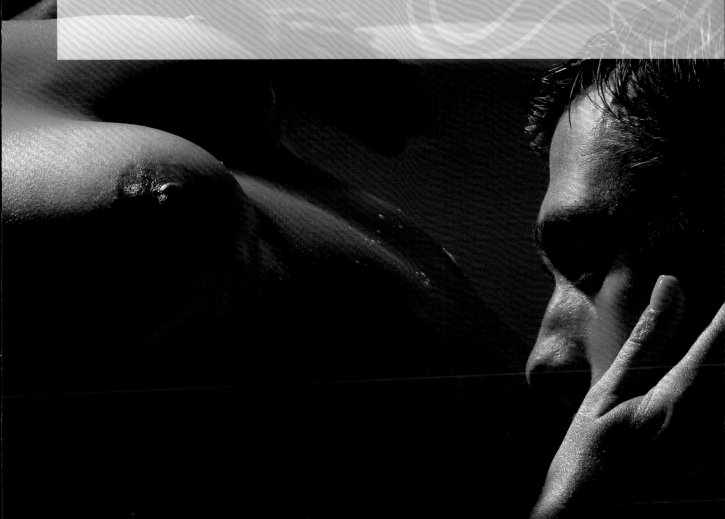

Chapter 5

Turning On in the Tub

PLEASURABLE TUB ACCOUTREMENTS

ALTHOUGH HAPPY ENDINGS are always optional, if you've gone to the trouble of prepping the room for a sensual bath, chances are good that it will culminate in some sort of pleasurable activity, whether you're alone or with a partner. Whether your pleasure is tantalizing or satisfying, the tub is the ideal environment for all things sexual.

AS SOME PEOPLE might already know, the tub and shower are already equipped for giving pleasure—if you know a few tricks. Lock the bathroom door, turn on some soothing tunes, and discover what your bathroom plumbing can do for *you*.

The Tap

Depending on what kind of faucet your tub has, it can be a source of extreme pleasure. The steady flow of water, whether dripping agonizingly slowly or streaming intensely, is a sublime sex toy women have been enjoying for decades. Position yourself so that your pelvis is directly under the faucet, and then adjust the water to the flow that best stimulates you.

Handheld Showerheads

Usually available with multispeed functions, a handheld showerhead is essential for any woman's bathroom. Shop around for a model that suits your bathroom's décor and fits easily in your hand. You'll want at least three functions: regular water pressure, a gentle massage function, and a "speed" or high-intensity massage function.

Play with the different functions of your shower-head to determine what feels good for you. Many women find the high-intensity massage spray to be too intense for direct clitoral stimulation, while others love a higher impact, pulsating-rhythm spray.

Try using the gentler settings for foreplay. First soothe your lover's aching muscles, and then aim a stream of water at his or her nipples. Work up to using the higher-intensity settings, using the firmest setting as he or she gets ready to climax.

European-style bathtubs are often equipped with a stationary tap in the middle of the tub, with a handheld showerhead resting next to it. Lying sideways in the tub, with your pelvis positioned under the tap and your legs propped on the wall behind the tub or resting over the edges of it, turn on the faucet and adjust the flow of water to your desired temperature and pressure. Allow the gentle dripping of warm water to stimulate your clitoris and labia while you or your partner uses the handheld showerhead's stream to titillate your other erogenous zones, such as your neck or nipples.

Toys

The sensual bath, already an erotically charged adventure, is made even more exotic with the addition of a toy or two. Whether using them alone or with a partner, sex toys were made for the bath—literally!

Waterproof sex toys are completely safe for fun in the tub, and are available in an incredibly diverse assortment of styles, designs, sizes, shapes, and colors. If you've never bought a sex toy before and are nervous about the experience, try shopping online. More experienced or adventurous people may prefer to shop for their toys in person. Visit www.goodvibrations.com or www.babeland.com for a variety of different sex toys.

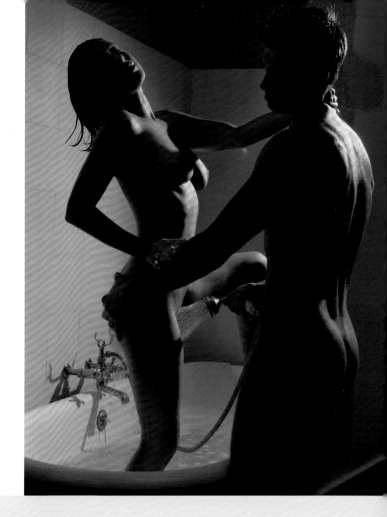

When I was a teenager, I discovered masturbation in the shower quite by accident. My dad had just installed a handheld showerhead in the bathroom, and while using it to rinse myself, a hard stream of water caught me between the legs in just the right spot. It felt strange and wonderful at the same time. After a few breathless minutes, I had my first orgasm.

—Annette, 26

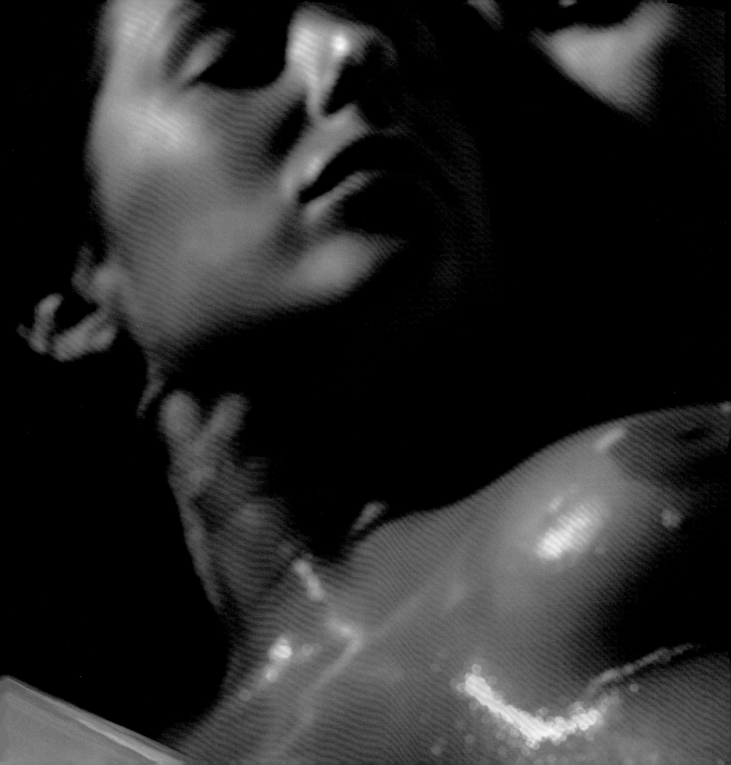

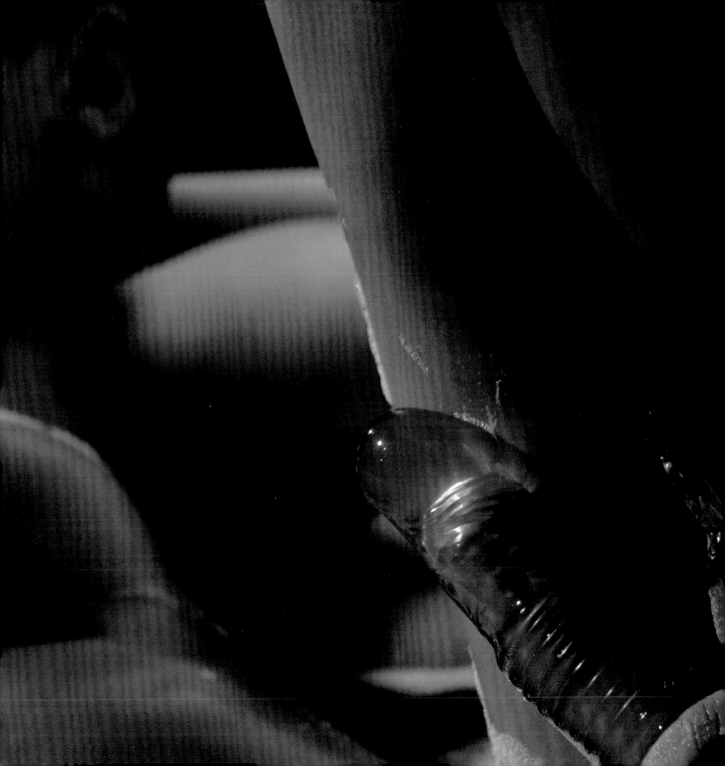

You'll need to keep a few things in mind when you use your sex toys in the bathtub. Water-based lube won't do the job, so make sure you use only silicone-based lube when playing in water. Also, if you plan to share your toy or interchange vaginal and anal use, always put a condom over the toy so that you don't inadvertently transmit bacteria from person to person (or orifice to orifice). Finally, always clean your toy after each use, dry it thoroughly, and store it in a dry place.

Waterproof Vibrators

Water and electricity might not mix, but water and battery-powered fun sure do. Whether you are using a vibe alone or with a partner, in the tub or in the shower, the sensation of intense vibration feels especially nice underwater.

Although waterproof vibrators can resemble anything from a lipstick to a kitty cat, most have one of four basic designs.

- **Traditional Vibrators**—Phallic in shape, traditional vibrators are designed primarily for vaginal use. Choose from a wide range of colors, sizes, and shapes, from realistic-looking to space-age. Waterproof materials range from hard plastic, which transmits powerful vibrations, to jelly and other "jiggly" materials, which feel lifelike and warm to the touch.
- **Clitoral Vibrators**—Designed to provide the kind of concentrated vibration women love, clitoral vibrators come in two forms. The mini vibrator—also known as the "pocket rocket"—

miniaturizes the concept of the vibrator, using hard plastic to transmit intense vibrations. The bullet consists of an oblong, vaguely egg-shaped vibrating bullet attached by a cord to a battery pack/controller, often featuring multiple speeds.

- **G-spot Vibrators**—Similar in appearance to traditional vibrators, these vibes have one noticeable difference: The tip is bent to apply pressure to the G-spot. Many women, especially those who have difficulty climaxing, go wild with the combination of thrusting, vibration, and G-spot pressure. Men can also use G-spot vibrators to apply pressure to their prostate gland, which often results in an explosive orgasm.
- **Rabbit Vibrators**—Combining the best elements of traditional, bullet and G-spot vibrators, rabbit vibes have been designed to ring all your bells at once. First coming to national attention when Charlotte tried one on the HBO series *Sex and the City*, rabbit vibes are phallic in shape, with a little stylized animal—usually a bunny rabbit with long, upright ears—perched just right for simultaneous vaginal and clitoral pleasure. Some models have a band of rotating beads that applies pressure to the G-spot. All these bells and whistles are controlled by a battery pack attached to the base of the vibrator with a cord. Many rabbit vibes have a multifunction controller that allows you to vary the speed and the type of stimulus: vibration, gyrating beads, and clitoral buzzing—or all three at once!

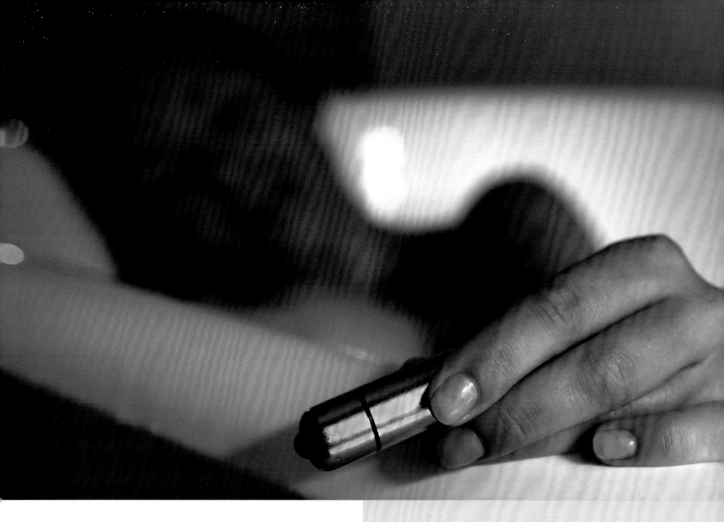

Of course, just because a waterproof vibrator was designed to stimulate a certain body part, that doesn't mean you can't use it on another! Bullet vibrators do wonderful things for nipples, be they male or female ones, and traditional vibrators feel lovely when traced gently over an erect penis. You can also use vibrating toys to relax the neck and shoulders and bring waves of pleasure to your erogenous zones.

Spice It Up

BUNNY BUZZ

Some people joke that a woman with a rabbit vibe doesn't need a man, but given all the permutations of speed and function, it's kind of nice to have an extra pair of hands, especially when you're nearing orgasm.

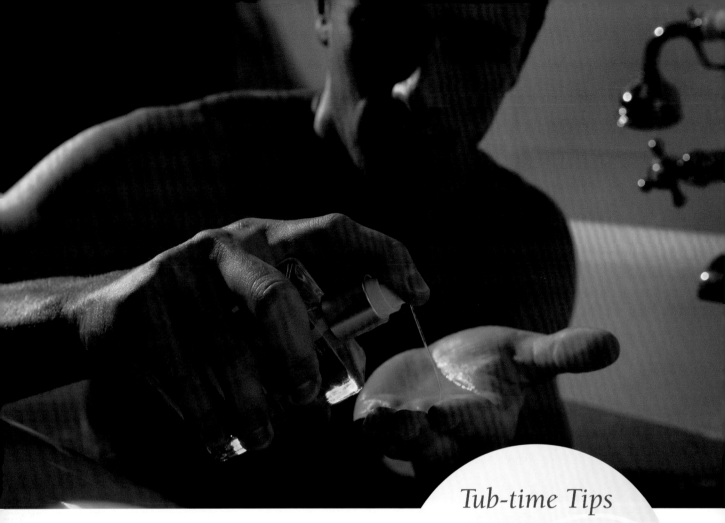

Waterproof Dildos

The general rule is that vibrators vibrate and dildos
don't. Many people, men and women alike, prefer
dildos to vibrators for vaginal and anal use. After all, it's
your body, and you know best what pleases it. If thrusting is for you, then so is a dildo.

Designed to provide pleasure through penetration,
the sensation of fullness and the application of
pressure, dildos are phallic in shape and usually made

Tub-time Tips

CHOOSING LUBE

Lubricant comes in three basic
forms: water-based, silicone-based, and
petroleum-based. Since water-based lube
washes off in water, it's a poor choice for
sensual bathing. Petroleum-based lubes
are too heavy and greasy to use in
the tub. Stick with a silicone-based
lube, which will last longer.

of a soft material around a firm base. Waterproof dildos are constructed of materials designed to last when the toy is used in water, even chlorinated Jacuzzi water and sudsy bathwater.

Care for your dildo the same way you'd care for your vibrator, by keeping it clean and using a condom on it if you plan to share it or swap it out between your front and backsides.

Other Tub Toys

If you find you like having a few grown-up toys in the tub, you'll be delighted to learn that adult toy designers have created a treasure trove of gadgets to take in the bath with you.

- **Waterproof Anal Toys**—Like their vaginal counterparts, waterproof anal toys are made in two basic varieties: vibrating and not vibrating. Men and women can enjoy both kinds of anal toys, especially in the shower, where everyone— and every body part—is a lot more relaxed.

- **Waterproof Erection Ring**—Designed to prolong a man's erection, these waterproof variants, usually made of pliable latex rubber or jelly, work well in the bath. Leave the metal and leather rings for use on dry land—neither are safe for use in water.

- **Waterproof Vibrating Couple's Ring**—Similar in design and function to the waterproof erection ring, the couple's ring gives pleasure to both partners. It's a simple design—the rubber ring stretches over the base of the penis, allowing the

Acoustics Alert!

As anyone who sings in the shower knows, your bathroom tile, especially in the tub or shower, makes any voice sound better—and louder. Keep your bathroom's acoustics in mind when using waterproof vibrators or any toy that makes noise. If you live alone, you may not care if your toy can be heard outside the bathroom, but people with roommates or children will want to be careful—even the quietest and most discreet vibrator can produce quite a racket in the tub.

The Glorious G-spot

Named after Ernst Grafenberg, the doctor who first wrote about this "erotic" area, the G-spot is located on the anterior wall of the vagina.

To find this elusive spot, insert your forefinger and middle finger into your vagina and make a "come hither" motion until you feel a patch of thick textured skin on the upper wall of your vagina, about the width of a quarter.

Once you've located the G-spot, experiment with applying differing levels of pressure. You may need lots of practice before you find the right touch for that magic button.

waterproof bullet to nestle against her clitoris. A variable-speed remote keeps her guessing what speed of pleasure will hit her next.

- **Grown-up Rubber Ducky**: This traditional-looking tub toy has a naughty little secret—it vibrates! Lull your lover into a state of total relaxation by massaging her back and shoulders, and then bring her to climax by using the toy as a clitoral vibrator.

Storing Your Toys

Although you might find it convenient to leave your toys in the shower caddy, next to the shampoo and body wash, you're probably better off storing them elsewhere. After cleaning your toys, drying them thoroughly, and removing any batteries, stash your toys in an airtight container in your bathroom cabinet, where they will be ready whenever you are.

My wife has always had a devil of a time climaxing during sex. Nothing worked until we tried a waterproof rabbit vibrator in a warm bubble bath. The combination of deep penetration, G-spot stimulation, and the intense vibrations the clitoral teaser transmits underwater are strong enough to bring her to a shattering orgasm almost every time!

—David, 42

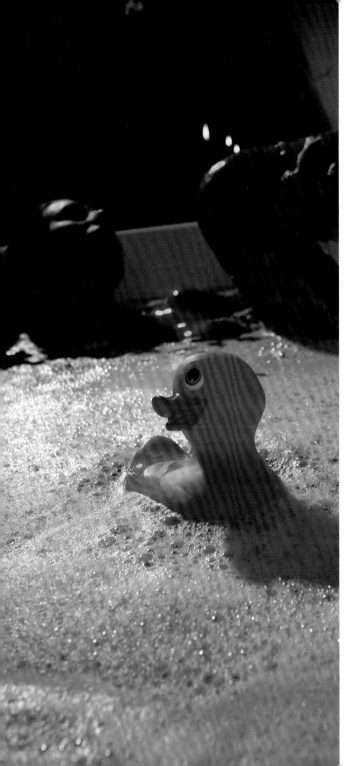

Making Waves

Including toys in your sensual bath experience can be a welcome addition, but before you run to grab all your old favorites there are some important things to consider.

Vibrator Safety Tips

Waterproof toys all have one factor in common: they are safe to use in the bath or shower (or hot tub or pool . . .). Use common sense and leave the non-waterproof toys in the bedroom, where they belong, and never, ever use toys powered by electricity in the tub. Getting electrocuted is not sexy.

Thicker Is Slicker

Many people find that dildos—especially those made of rubber and realistic materials—chafe a bit after a little thrusting. Opt for a thicker waterproof lube, such as those formulated for anal play, and your dildo will stay smooth and slick. Just make sure your lube is chemically compatible with your dildo; petroleum lubes destroy most sex toys.

Cleaning Waterproof Toys

Waterproof toys—no matter what material they're made of—are easier to clean than most other sex toys. All you'll need to do is run them under warm water and voilà—that's it! If you have a large collection of toys, you can even run them through the dishwasher; just skip the soap, which can damage some toys.

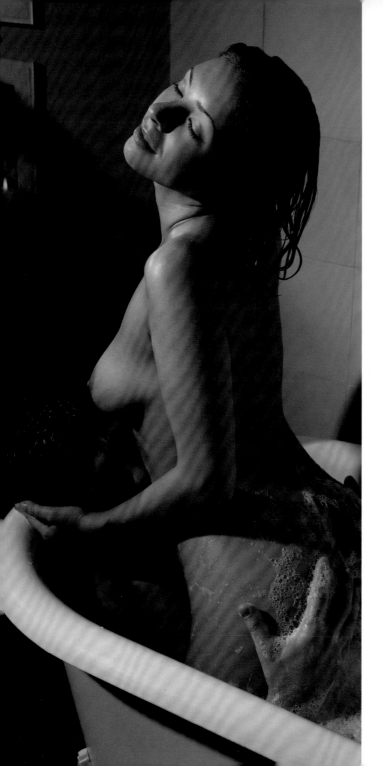

GETTING DIRTY

WHETHER YOU'RE A NEW COUPLE, still basking in the early days of your relationship, or one that has been together for many years, adding some kinky activity to spice up your sex life is a pretty natural progression for many couples. Taking this erotic behavior to the bathtub makes it even steamier!

Oral Play

The bathtub is a perfect location for both giving and receiving oral sex. After soaping up and rinsing off, your bodies will be squeaky-clean, alleviating any worries either partner may have about unpleasant tastes or odors. You and your partner may have to experiment a little before you find the position that works best for you—the receiving partner leaning against the wall while the other partner sits on the edge of the tub; or the receiving partner sitting on the edge of the tub while the other partner sits or kneels in the tub. A folded towel under each knee will make the experience more comfortable!

Anal Play

Although anal play doesn't appeal to everyone, many people find it incredibly erotic. Part of the excitement stems from our perception of anything anal as taboo—things that are naughty or forbidden are often downright sexy. Ultimately, though, anal play can be quite pleasurable! Our buttocks, anus, and rectum contain millions of nerve endings, which respond well to all kinds of stimulation. Men are also blessed with

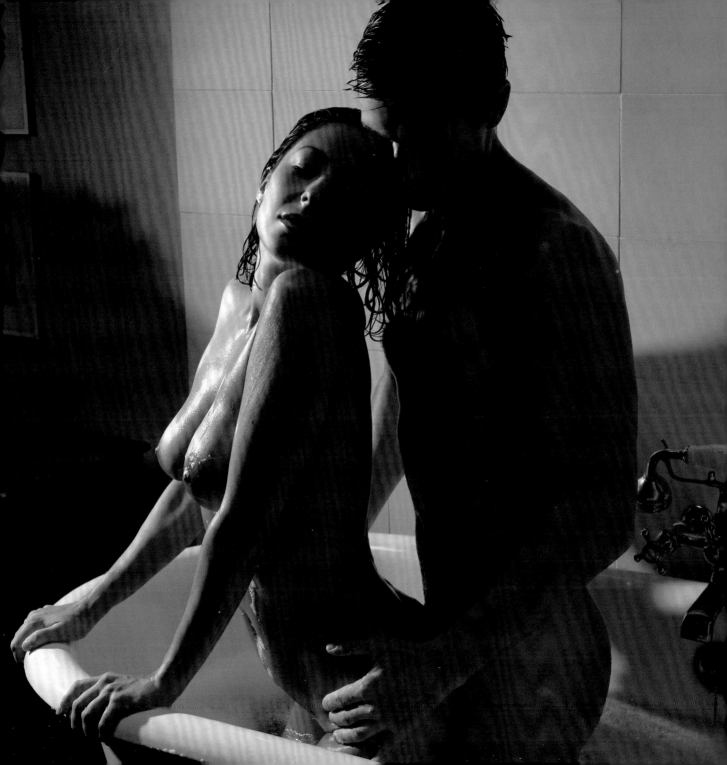

the prostate gland. In addition to serving the biological purpose of helping create semen, the prostate feels intensely aroused when stimulated with firm pressure.

If you have been fantasizing about anal play but are still uncomfortable with the idea, the tub is a great place to explore this form of sexual expression, alone or with a partner. With lots of soap and water at hand, you won't have to worry about the "dirty parts" of anal play. Also, the combination of hot water and sensuality create an atmosphere in which you and your partner might feel ready to try things previously unexplored.

Try using the faucet or handheld shower head to stimulate the sensitive skin around your anus. Men can aim the water a little deeper, using harder pressure, for prostate stimulation. Because hot water can dry out delicate skin, don't engage in this form of play for more than 20 to 30 minutes.

Getting Kinky with Fantasy Play

If you and your partner enjoy a little game of "let's pretend" in the boudoir, try moving your fantasy play into the bath. As the hot water steams open your pores, it will also relax your mind, making you agreeable to experiences you might not otherwise want to try.

Light bondage and domination can turn your tame ablutions into a seriously erotic encounter. Try blindfolding or restraining your partner during a sensual bath by removing power from one partner and placing it entirely with another. By relinquishing power, you surrender a little something of yourself for the duration of your encounter, elevating your play to new heights of sensuality.

You might also try spanking your lover in the shower. Be sure to discuss this first! Spanking doesn't appeal to everyone. However, those that enjoy the gentle warming of

My boyfriend, Sam, and I have always enjoyed bathing together and playing with sex toys during our lovemaking. Most recently he tried out a new remote controlled cock ring on me. I didn't realize he was wearing the toy until he entered me. At first, all I could feel was a little extra padding around the base of his penis, but then he used the remote control to buzz my clitoris while thrusting into me. The pleasure was so intense that I almost screamed!

—Lorraine, 41

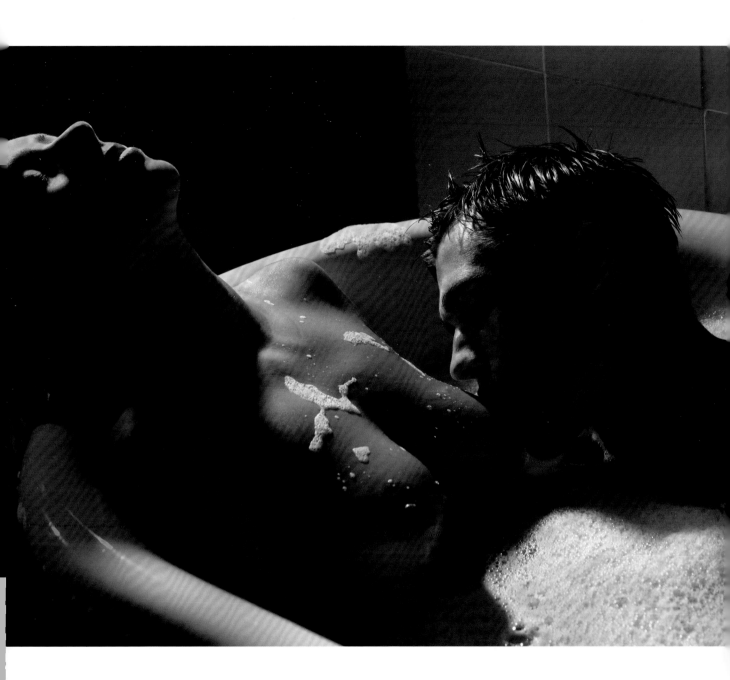

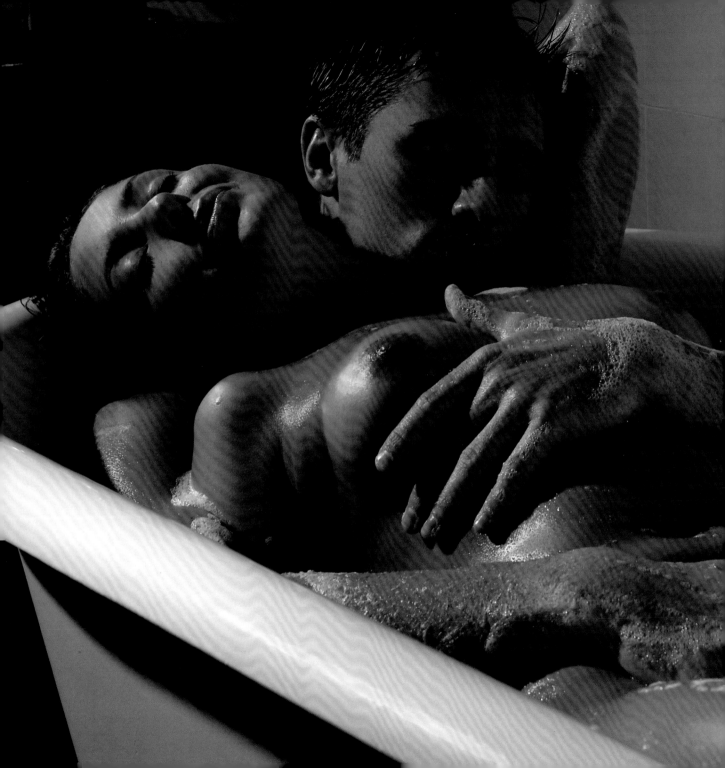

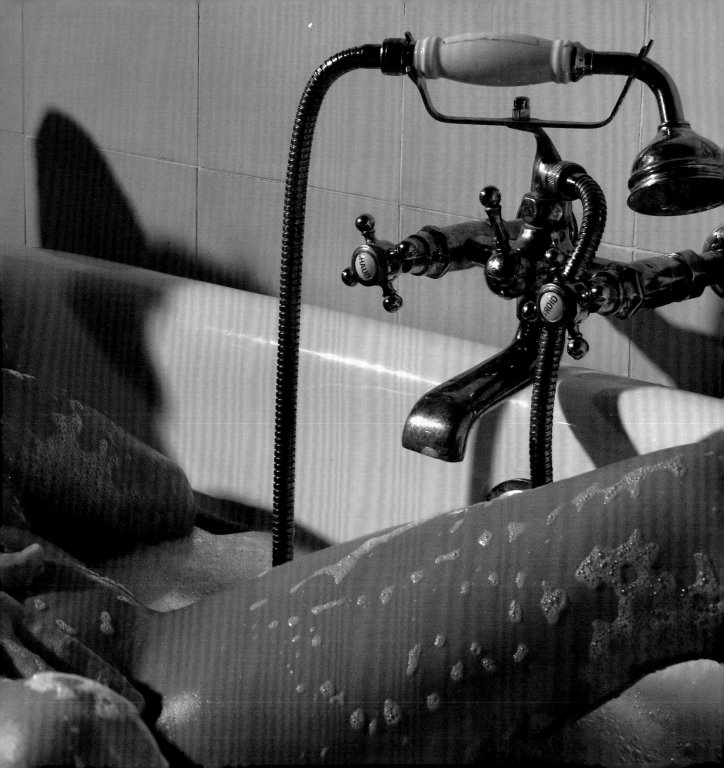

Pick a Safe Word

Before you and your partner engage in any kind of new sexual activity, have an honest discussion about your desires. It might be an awkward conversation to initiate, but it will be a lot more comfortable than trying something without knowing whether or not your partner is agreeable. Once you get the green light, you and your partner should pick a "safe word," a word or phrase you'd otherwise never say during a romantic encounter, such as "apple" or "chair." When someone utters the safe word, the play stops immediately.

spanked buttocks will love what water adds to the experience, especially when light bondage is involved.

Fetishes are forms of sexual play that some people might consider weird or "abnormal." However, as long as you aren't breaking the law or hurting anyone—including yourself!—there is nothing wrong with exploring your fascination with activities or accoutrements not traditionally considered erotic. Some common fetishes include licking women's feet or cross dressing—wearing clothing meant for the opposite sex.

Because of its proximity to large quantities of soap and water, the tub is a natural location for many kinds of fetish play. The physically relaxing atmosphere of the sensual bath can also steam open minds, yours or your partners, enabling you to feel comfortable with new forms of erotic play.

Tub-time Tips

SKID-PROOF LOVE
Even when warm, porcelain isn't very comfortable. Cushion your backside with a towel or tub mat, and use a bath pillow to cushion and elevate your head.

Dennis and I *love to explore our fantasies in the bathtub. The bathroom is our "secret place," where we experiment with our deepest desires. A long time ago, we made a pact that what we do in the bath stays in the bath, which only heightens the arousal and excitement for both of us. We both get the most pleasure when he spanks me with his bare hand, but we've had fun with some props, too.*

—Debbie, 43

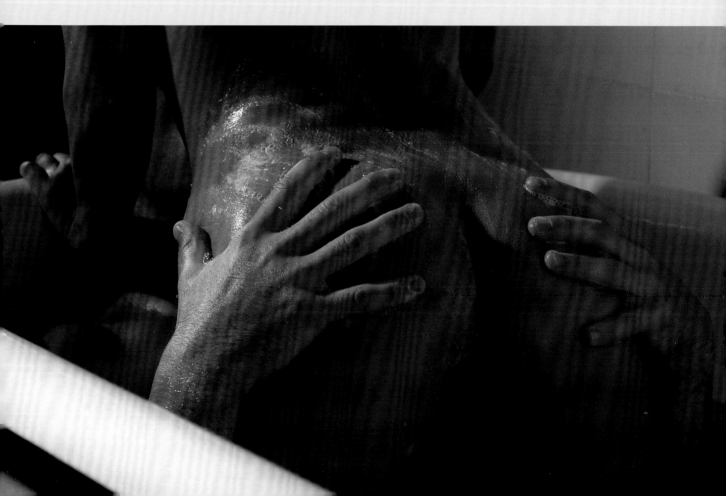

Chapter 6

The Solo Sensual Bath

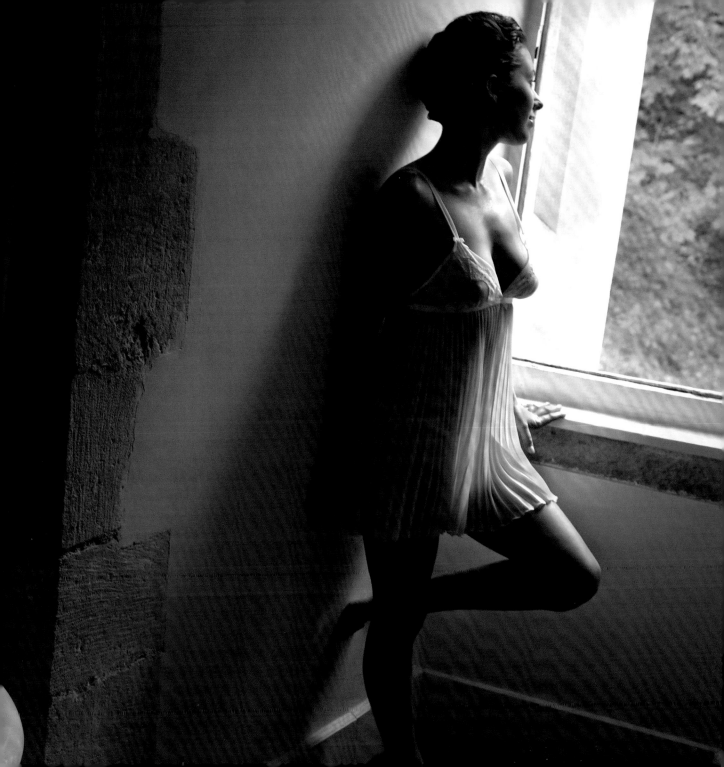

SOLITARY SEDUCTION

EVEN IF YOUR GOAL isn't having an orgasm, your body, mind, and spirit will benefit from the invigorating relaxation you'll experience with a sensual bath.

WHEN DRAWING A BATH FOR YOURSELF, take the time to create a space that appeals to your specific senses and personal ideas about sensuality.

Clean your tub and bathroom and set out freshly laundered towels. Draw yourself a bath, adding a few drops of your favorite essential oils. Light a few candles, perhaps some incense, and place a cold bottle of water and a bouquet of fresh flowers on a chair or stool next to the tub. Turn off the bathroom lights—and your cell phone!—and slip into the tub, allowing the warm water to cover as much of your body as possible.

Close your eyes, drape a wet washcloth over them, and take a few moments to relax, allowing your breathing to slow and deepen as each muscle in your body relaxes.

Pampering Yourself

The time for pampering is now, before you start thinking sexy thoughts. Use a loofah and a rich body wash to cleanse and exfoliate your skin. Shampoo and condition your hair, shave if you need to—you can even enjoy a skin or hair treatment.

As you care for yourself, pay attention to the way your hands feel on your body. Bask in the sensuality you experience when you take the time to really clean and pamper yourself. When you're done, drain the tub, rinsing yourself completely, from head to toe. Refill the tub with clean, warm water, adding more oils if you'd like.

Seducing Yourself

It might feel silly at first, but there is no reason to forego foreplay when bathing solo. You might be tempted to skip ahead to the main event, but taking the time to kindle and stoke your desire will yield the same payoff as extended partner foreplay: stronger, longer, more satisfying orgasms. And really, who *doesn't* want that?

The fastest way to rev your libido is to take some erotica into the tub with you, whether it is a book or magazine (keep a towel nearby in case you accidentally splash the pages). You can also replay your favorite fantasy or create a new one—do whatever it takes to get your party started.

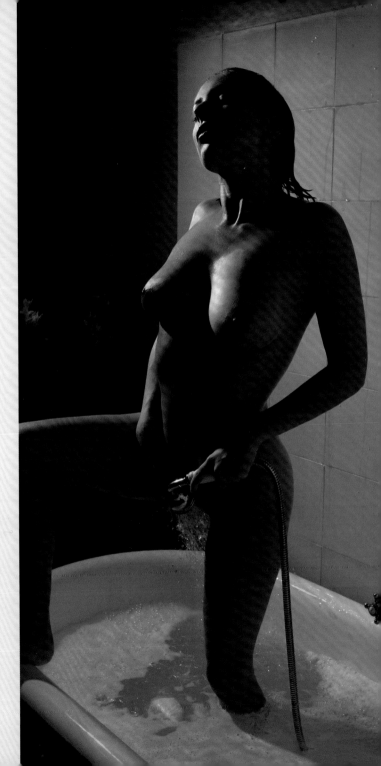

Soothing Your Mind

If you find it difficult to stop worrying
about problems and fretting over
tasks still undone, try a relaxation
exercise to empty your mind of
unpleasant thoughts. Close your eyes
and visualize a blank piece of paper.
Take no more than one minute to
mentally jot down a list of your
worries. Once the page is filled,
picture an invisible hand folding the
paper into a tiny square. Visualize
yourself placing the paper square in a
safe place, preferably in another
room. Give yourself permission to
think about your problems after your
bath, when your refreshed and
relaxed body, mind, and spirit may
give you a different perspective.

As you begin to feel aroused, use your free hand to squeeze warm water from a sponge onto the exposed parts of your body. Let your hand wander, down your throat, over your chest, and play with your nipples, just as a lover would do. Graze the sensitive skin of your inner thighs with your nails. Tease yourself a little, allowing your fingers to dip between your legs without lingering too long. Take your time and enjoy the sensations you are experiencing.

SENSUAL SELF-PLEASURE

EVEN IF YOU'VE BEEN MASTURBATING for years—and most people *have*, by the way, regardless of what they might claim—touching yourself in the tub might be a totally new experience for you. Everything feels different when water is involved, so enjoy this chance to find out what turns you on.

Self-pleasuring for Her

Self-love is exactly that: the opportunity to love your body in exactly the way that feels best to *you*. Unfortunately, many women have difficulty climaxing during partner sex, so masturbation is an excellent way of discovering how your body responds to different sexual stimulation.

As you become more comfortable and aroused, set down your book, close your eyes, and let your fingers do the walking. Begin slowly and vary the speed and intensity until your body responds with a loud "Yes!"

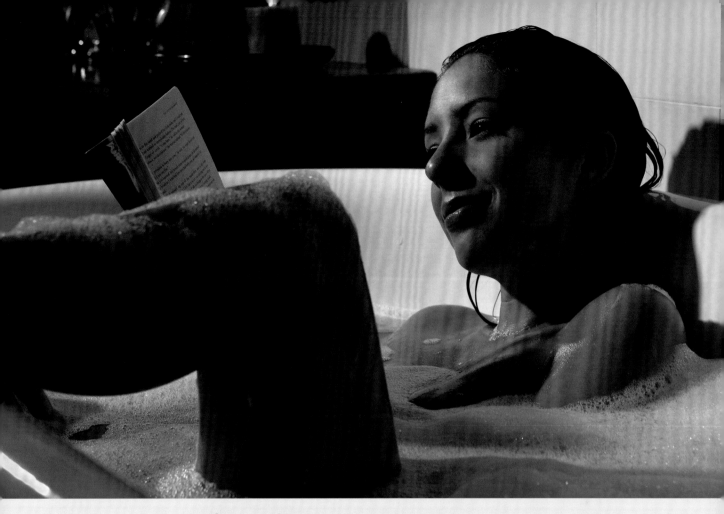

After soaking in a tub full of hot, fragrant water, my mind wanders to the lustful, especially if I'm reading erotica. Slipping a warm washcloth over my forehead, I close my eyes and recline in the tub. With one heel on the edge of the tub, I tilt my pelvis upward, meeting my hands. Sighing, I surrender to pleasure.

—*Alexis, 29*

It might take some time and practice, but with diligence, you'll be an expert in no time. Don't be afraid to try new things—you might discover something your partner will be delighted to try on you later.

While you're searching out new places that delight you underwater, try a few moves with which you might not be acquainted:

- With your index finger, trace the alphabet or "count" to 50 on your clitoris. You probably won't climax with this move, but you will discover some new sensations worth repeating.

- Place two fingers directly on your clitoris and move them in a circular motion, varying your speed and pressure.

- Place your thumb and forefinger on either side of your clitoris and gently roll it between your fingertips. If direct clitoral stimulation is too intense for you, try the same movement just above your clitoris.

- Lightly draw a spiral around your vulva, working in smaller concentric circles until you are gently circling your clitoris with your middle finger. Spiral back out and in as your pleasure dictates, varying your speed as your climax builds.

- While gently rubbing your clitoris with one hand, use your other hand to insert a few fingers into your vagina, simulating the thrusting of inter-course. Many women don't realize how exciting the combination of penetration and clitoral stimulation can be until they try it for themselves, and what better place to try than the tub?

- Enhance your experience with a waterproof sex toy. Water transmits vibrations in a very different way from what you experience when using your toys in the boudoir. Many women find anal toys a welcome addition during masturbation—you'll never know if you don't try it.

MASTURBATION IS FOR YOU and you alone, so take your time and enjoy yourself. During your time in the tub, you are the only person you need to please. If you don't feel like having an orgasm, you don't have to. With all the sensitive skin and nerve endings between your legs you're going to have a good time, regardless of the outcome

Tub-time Tips

WATER WON'T KEEP YOU WET
Sensitive flesh does not respond well when moistened with nothing but water. Use a silicone-based lube when you're masturbating in the tub. Men will find the slippery sensation of lube and water quite erotic, and women, whose natural lubrication doesn't last long in a warm bath, will feel smooth and silky, even after 15 minutes.

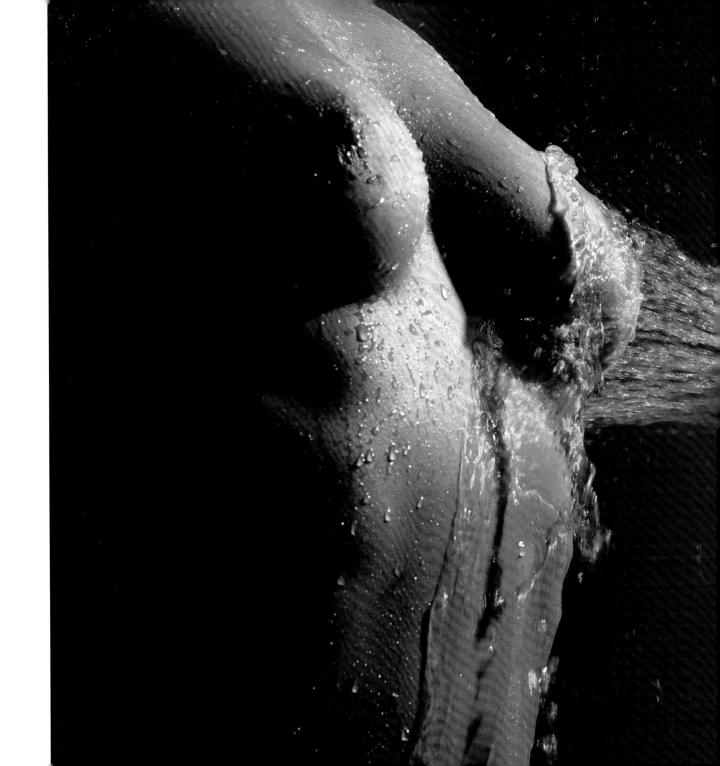

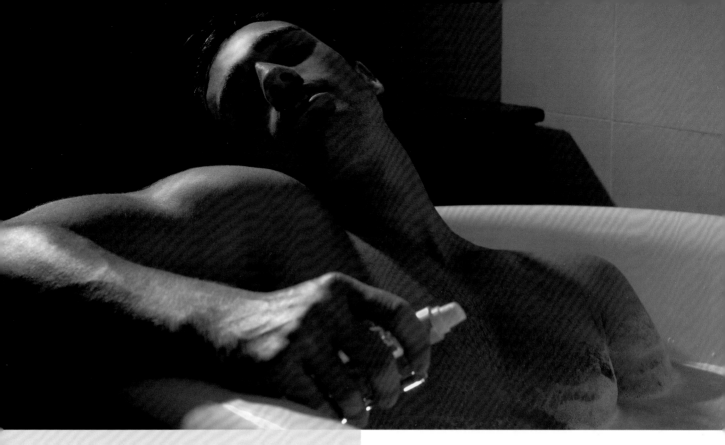

Spice It Up

SLAP YOURSELF SILLY

Slap your penis around a little. Before you start to climax, when your penis is hard and super-sensitive, gently slap it from side to side with your open palm. You might also graze the sensitive underside with your fingernails. Be gentle: the object is not pain, but pleasure.

Self-pleasuring for Him

Although most men are quite adept at pleasuring themselves, even the classic move—wrapping your fingers around your erect penis and stroking it up and down until you ejaculate—can feel entirely different during a sensual bath. There's something about the combination of a steam-filled room, a tub full of warm water, and the slippery friction produced by silicone lube and water. Enjoy the way your favorite moves feel underwater, or try something new.

• The simplest variation is using your non-dominant hand to masturbate. As you stroke yourself, you can imagine your hand belongs to someone gorgeous and naked.

- Use both hands at once, one at the base of your penis and one at the head. Slide your hands up and down your shaft in a pumping motion, or gently twist both hands in opposite directions.

- With one hand, stroke your penis from its head to its base, releasing it when you reach your scrotum. Meanwhile, perform the same motion with your other hand, alternating hands and strokes, one after the other, developing a rhythm.

- Make a circle of your thumb and forefinger and squeeze the head of your penis through it, stroking the circle up and down your shaft. Try this same move with your hand held in a fist.

- Stroke only your shaft, ignoring the head of your penis, which will swell and become incredibly sensitive. When your penis is fully erect, use your other hand to gently squeeze the head.

The Mysterious "Male G-spot"

The prostate is a small gland, about the size and shape of a small egg, which excretes the seminal fluid that helps guide sperm to their biological target. Nestled in the man's pubic bone and surrounded by the pelvic muscles, the prostate gland responds—usually very positively!—to pressure applied through the rectum. Prostate toys make this job easier, as do women's G-spot toys. Just make sure you select a toy with a flared base.

Once a week or so, I take my time in the shower and romance myself a little before masturbating. It helps me reconnect with my body—as I lather up, I take pleasure in the way my skin feels under my fingers. Touching my body in the shower allows me to enjoy all that hard work I do at the gym, and in turn, I feel sexier and more sensual.

—*Anthony, 21*

You may want to enhance your experience by using a waterproof erection ring, which will delay your orgasm and increase sensitivity, especially at the head of your penis. A vibrating ring used underwater transmits waves of pleasure along your shaft.

Although most men masturbate in order to have an orgasm, there's no need to rush. The point of treating yourself to a sensual bath is to relax and enjoy yourself. If you want to get down-and-dirty, take a shower!

POST-PLEASURE PAMPERING

JUST AS IN PARTNER SEX, men and women can both benefit from taking a few moments to bask in the afterglow of their solo sensual baths. Before you drain the bath and put away the toys, end your night on a positive note by pampering yourself just a little longer.

Dry your body with a plush towel, preferably an oversized bath sheet made from Egyptian or Turkish cotton. Use a rich, creamy moisturizer on your hands, feet, and body. Put on fresh, clean clothing or pajamas (or nothing at all!), and slip your feet into cozy slippers.

Ease yourself back into the real world a bit at a time, taking tasks slowly and waiting until the last possible second to turn on the lights. Reality will soon be upon you, so savor these last few moments of totally *you* time.

One evening while soaking in the tub, I spied the little Aqua Vibe a friend had given me for my last birthday. I'd stashed it with my other shower accessories, but I hadn't yet used it. I fished it out of the shower caddy and when I touched it to my clitoris, it was like a tidal wave crashed over me, the vibrations were that strong. After the blinding orgasm I had that day, the Aqua Vibe became my best bath-time buddy.

—Michelle, 38

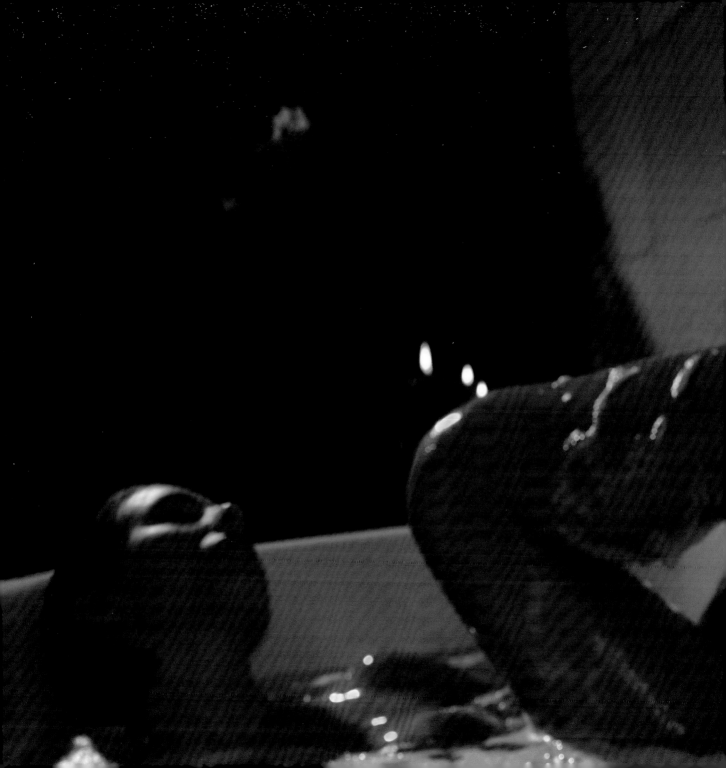

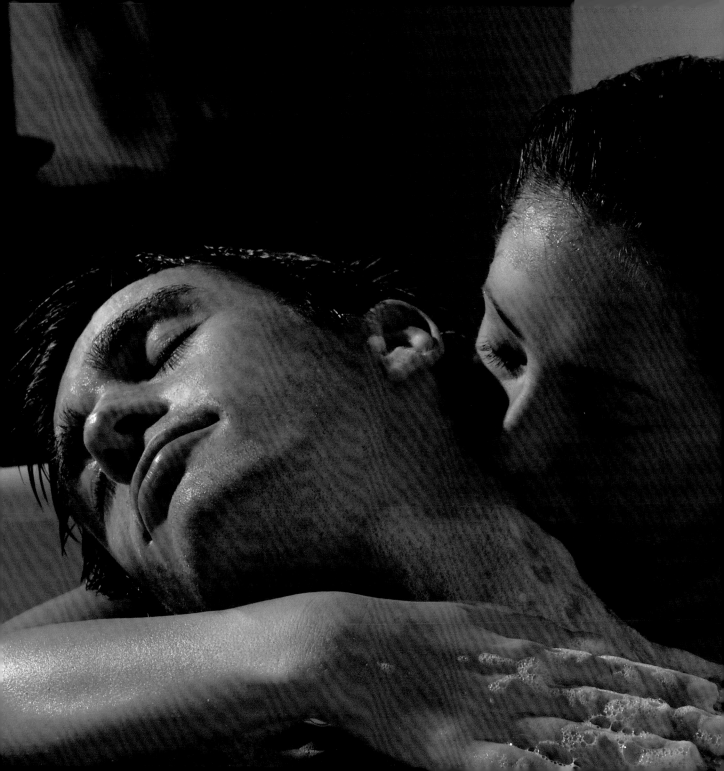

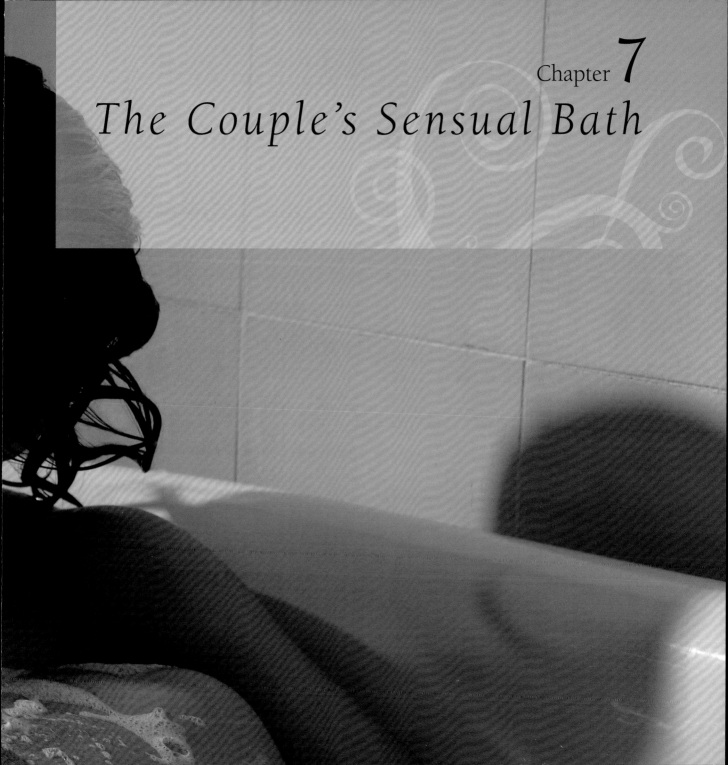

Chapter 7

The Couple's Sensual Bath

SHARING EROTIC INTIMACY

SHARING A SENSUAL BATH with your partner is about much more than getting clean or getting down-and-dirty. Enjoy the time you spend together in the bath, and learn what pleases your partner best. Caring for one another is a very special form of intimacy that strengthens and deepens the bond between two people.

WHEN CREATING A SENSUAL SPACE for yourself and your partner, take special care to incorporate elements that appeal to both of you. Until you determine your own preferences, experiment with different combinations to set the mood.

Saucy and Playful

To release inhibitions and create an atmosphere of openness and comfort, keep the mood lively and light. This combination is perfect for beginners.

- Place a bouquet of fresh sunflowers or brightly colored gerbera daisies in several vases around the room. Use incense or an oil burner to infuse the air with fruity, floral scents, like bergamot, orange, cinnamon, or geranium.
- Place a bowl of fresh, sliced fruit and carafe of chilled white wine near the tub.
- Purchase fun, comfortable his-and-hers pajamas, launder them, and set them in the bathroom to wear when you're dry again.
- Play fun music like Pink Martini, the Beatles, Belle and Sebastian, or the Polyphonic Spree.
- Light a dozen bright yellow and orange candles, placing them around the room. Although you don't want the bright glare of the overhead light, keep the room fairly well lit.

Romantic

Woo your partner with a soft touch, incorporating traditionally romantic elements into your sensual bath.

- Adorn the room with small bouquets of red and pink roses. Infuse the air with a scent of jasmine, preferably in the form of oil simmering in a burner.
- Select several large, juicy strawberries with the stems still attached. Warm a small dish of chocolate sauce to accompany the berries. Uncork a bottle of champagne or sparkling wine, and keep it on ice.
- Fill the bath with warm water softened with aromatic bath oil. Scatter a few rose petals on the water.
- Select your partner's favorite love songs or play classical music—skip anything overly bombastic. Sade, Barry White, or other smooth jazz is another good choice.
- Light three or four large white pillar candles. If your bathroom lacks visual appeal, experiment with draping sheer scarves or fabric over the windows to create instant romance.

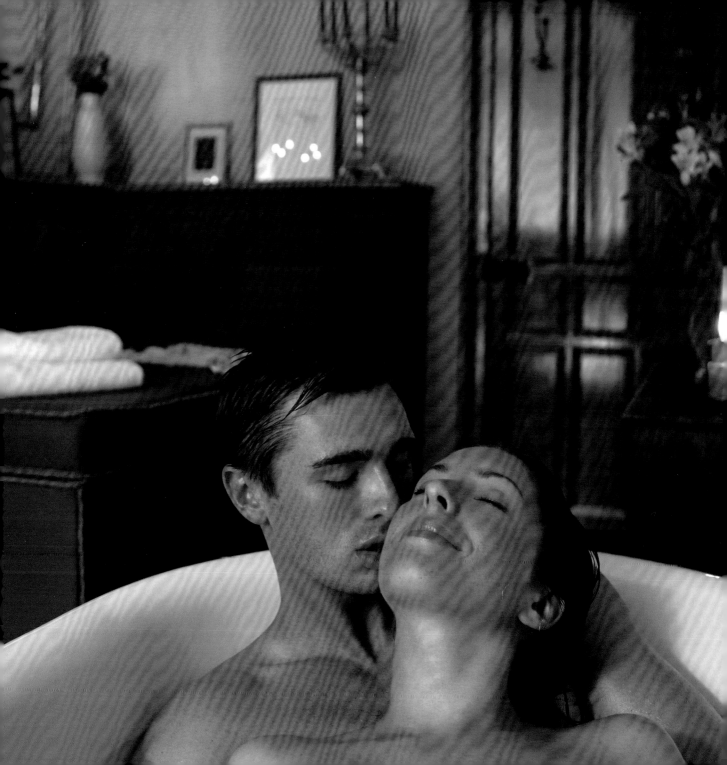

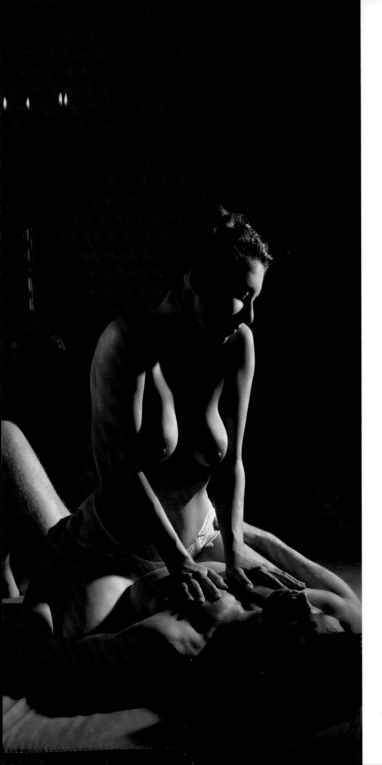

Seductive

When your goal is straightforward seduction, pull out all the stops to create a dramatic, sensual room.

- Create a bouquet of a single kind of visually interesting flower, such as bird-of-paradise, tuberose, lilies, or black roses. Infuse the room with exotic, spicy fragrances, like jasmine, sandalwood, or patchouli.
- Set out a tray of dark chocolate, raspberries, and red wine. If neither of you has a sweet tooth, try shelled nuts, flavorful cheese, and cognac or brandy. Limit heartier fare to shrimp cocktail or raw oysters.
- Select an assortment of sensual props, such as whipped cream, a blindfold, light restraints, and a bowl of ice. Even if you don't wind up using all your props, the sight of them will be exciting.
- Play intense, passionate music, like the Tindersticks, the soundtrack from *The Hunger*, or Chris Armstrong's *The Space Between Us*.
- To really make an impact, fill the room with dark red, purple, and black candles in a variety of sizes and shapes.
- Soften the bathwater with almond oil and six drops of a single, intense scent, like patchouli or ylang-ylang.

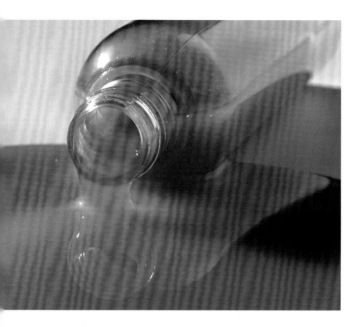

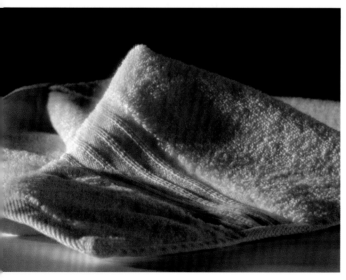

SENSUAL SHOPPING LIST

No matter what scenario you choose, you'll want to keep a few basic supplies on hand:

- **Silicone-based Lubricant**—Water-based lube washes right off, so select a lube with staying power.

- **Massage Oil**—Even the stickiest oil won't stand up to the shower spray, so feel free to experiment with different scents, textures, and consistencies. When you find one—or more—that appeals to you and your partner, stock up.

- **Bath Towels**—Select soft, plush, oversized linens in durable fabrics, like Egyptian or Turkish cotton.

SEDUCING YOUR LOVER

WHETHER THIS IS YOUR FIRST or fortieth sensual bath with your partner, begin the event properly by seducing your lover. Although you will best know what appeals to both of you, you might try to mix things up with something new.

Secret Seduction

Leave a series of clues for your lover to discover during the day. A note slipped into a handbag or briefcase could hint at something wet and wild, and a few strategic e-mail or voicemail messages can stoke the fire. At home, tape directions to the door and hallway, directing your partner to the bathroom, where you are waiting in the shower.

Seduce with a Gift

Surprise your partner with a gift—a new waterproof sex toy, a bottle of luxurious bath oil, a plush new bath towel—with instructions that it must be used *immediately*. You might even arrange to have the gift sent to your lover at work; just make sure the packaging is discreet!

Blind Seduction

Blindfold your partner and lead him or her to the bathroom. Leaving the blindfold in place, remove your lover's clothing and help him or her step into the tub. Before you remove the blindfold, spend a few minutes pampering your partner, teasing him or her with warm water squeezed from a sponge.

Seduce with a Striptease

Perform a slow, sensual striptease for your lover, forcing him to sit in place—no touching!—while you remove each article of clothing. When you're completely nude, remove his clothing, using your teeth whenever possible.

DOING ALL THE WORK all the time is no fun, so take turns seducing each other. As you and your partner discover what pleases you best in the bath, incorporate elements from different scenarios so that one of you always has the element of surprise to aid in the seduction.

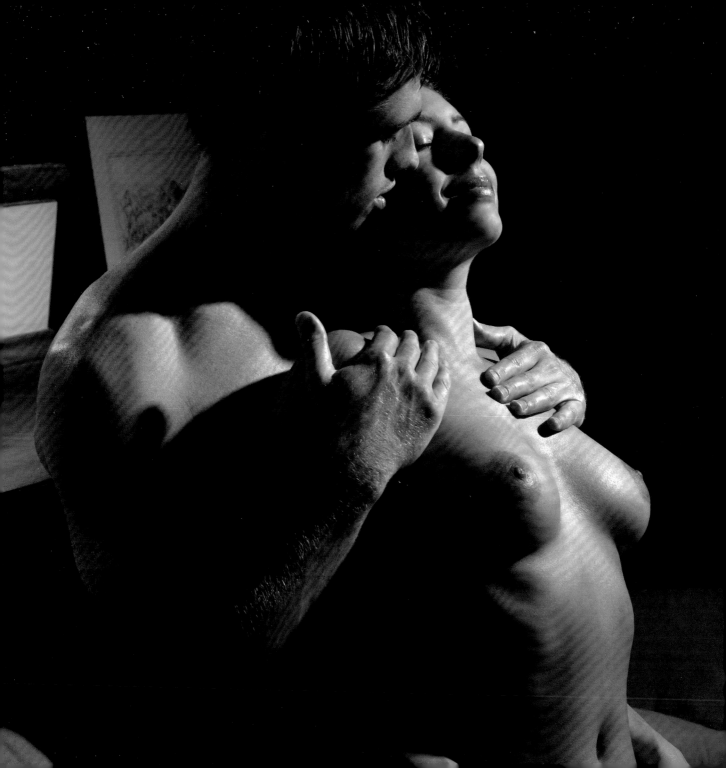

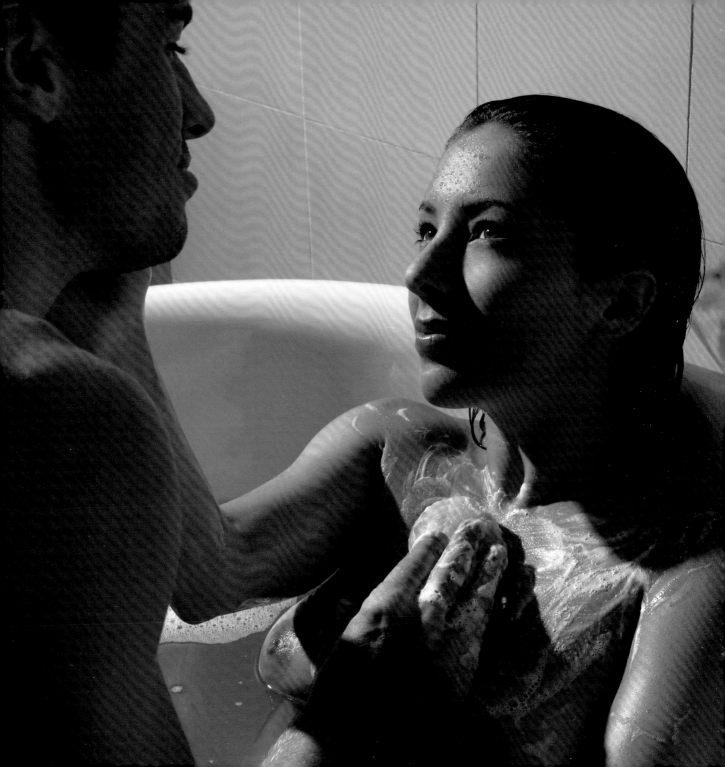

PAMPERING EACH OTHER

BEFORE DRAWING THE BATH water, shower together and cleanse yourselves. Use a large sponge and aromatic body wash—eucalyptus is unisex and invigorating, and not antiseptic or bracing—to lather each other. Shampoo, condition, and rinse each other's hair. As you and your partner pamper one another, enjoy the feelings of intimacy and trust you are building.

Shaving Together

Aside from the practical aspects of shaving together—touching up the bikini area is easier when someone else does it—many couples find that shaving one another not only brings a new level of intimacy to the relationship, but also serves as a sublime form of foreplay. If you're both amenable, take turns shaving each other's legs, face, and armpits. Adventurous couples might even try shaving one another between the legs.

When you think about it, allowing someone else to use a razor on your body requires a great deal of closeness. Entrusting your partner with this task shows that you are confident he or she will take care of you and treat your body with respect. For most people, that's a huge turn-on!

Whether you want smooth legs or a Brazilian, observe a few rules for the ultimate in a clean, nick-free shave:

- Always use a new blade, especially when your partner shaves you. The very last thing you want is a nick from a dull, rusty blade.
- Don't reach for the razor the second you turn on the water. Steam needs a few minutes to work, opening your pores and allowing for the blade to cut hair closer to the follicle. The result: a smoother shave that lasts longer.
- Use a thick, foamy cream to lather up before you shave. In a pinch, hair conditioner will do, as will regular body lotion. Rinse the razor after every stroke.
- Use downward strokes to shave; never go against the hair or your lover may get a red, bumpy rash—decidedly un-sexy, especially if you're shaving down below!

Make sure that you and your partner both have the same idea of what's going to happen. Going straight for the groin is not the smoothest of moves, especially when your partner has smooth pits in mind.

FOREPLAY: WET AND WILD

JUST AS YOU WOULD in bed, take time to work your lover into a frenzy before going for the gold. Although your technique will differ depending on the situation and mood, a few elements will work in almost any situation.

Make erotica part of your ritual while soaking in the bath. Lean back against your lover while you take turns reading aloud from your favorite "dirty" book. The sound of your lover's voice can be very sexy, even more so when he's reading erotic writing. The intimate act of experiencing erotica together will bring you and your partner closer—both emotionally and sexually!—strengthening the bond between you.

As you and your partner naturally escalate the heat between you, raise the stakes by using the massage feature on your handheld showerhead to stimulate your partner's erogenous zones.

Since this is still only foreplay, avoid too much genital contact. Focus on less-traveled areas, such as the back of the neck, the scalp, the bottoms of the feet, the underarms, and the nipples. Tease your lover, aiming the nozzle in unexpected patterns: scalp to nipples, belly to instep, buttocks to calves. Keep your partner guessing, and the anticipation will electrify your lovemaking.

Dirty Books for Good, Clean Fun

It's a fact: Unlike men, women respond better to the written word than they do to sexual images. If your partner happens to be a woman, you might want to invest in a few good erotic books:

- *Five-Minute Erotica*: Editor Carol Queen's short-short stories are the perfect length for reading aloud to a lover in the bath.

- *Down and Dirty: 69 Super Sexy Short-Shorts*: Even briefer—and more direct—is Alison Tyler's collection of quickie erotica.

- The *Sleeping Beauty* trilogy: Explore spanking, orgies, and adventurous forms of sexual play with this well-written series of books from vampire author Anne Rice.

- *Best Women's Erotica 2007*: Edited by Violet Blue, this collection of short stories spans a wide range of erotic encounters.

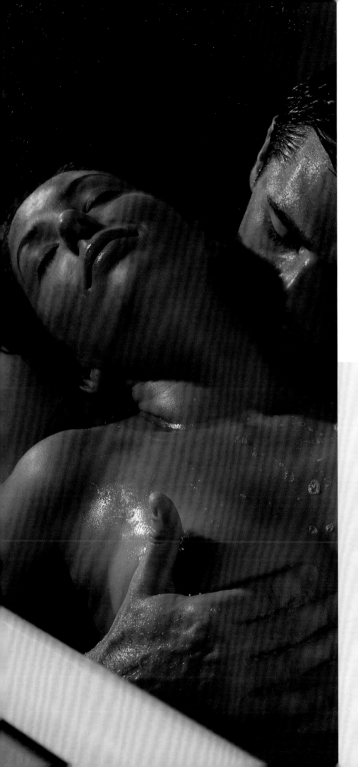

Even though you aren't quite ready to escalate the action, you can still energize your foreplay with a few sex toys. Use a waterproof vibrator to caress your partner's neck and shoulders, nipples, and belly. Although you might feint at genital contact, keep in mind that foreplay happens *before* the sex part!

When you and your partner reach a heightened state of arousal, you're ready to get to the good stuff—but first, prolong the ecstasy just a little longer by treating your lover to a sensual massage.

Spice It Up

TEASE AND TANTALIZE

Use the lightest grazing of your finger-nails to caress your lover's back, arms, and chest. Up the ante by stroking his or her belly, hips, buttocks and inner thighs, nearing—but not quite touching—the genitalia. The longer you tease your lover, the more excited you will both become; holding back often leads to explosive sex.

Bathtub Games

Add a playful note to your foreplay with a few simple lovers' games. The object is not to win, but to pleasure your lover in new ways.

- **Unseen Seduction**—Your lover reclines in the tub, a wet washcloth draped over his eyes, while you tease him with different sensations: a necklace pulled over his soapy chest, a comb traced over the sensitive flesh of her inner thighs, or cotton balls lightly brushing his nipples. Your partner's task it to guess what you're using to tantalize him.

- **Secret Message**—On your partner's soapy back, trace a short love note, such as "Take me," "I love you" or "You taste delicious," while your partner tries to guess what you're scribbling. To add incentive, you might also try writing directions for pleasing you.

- **Favorite Fantasy**—Take turns acting out your fantasies. One night, he could be a pirate king ravishing the governor's daughter; the next, she could be a lusty barmaid to his wandering minstrel.

SENSUAL MASSAGE FOR THE BATH

POUR ABOUT TWO tablespoons of massage oil into the palm of your hand, and rub them together lightly, warming the oil. Try to distribute the oil evenly over your palms and fingers. Your hands should be coated with just a thin layer of oil, not dripping with it.

Keep the massage oil handy and reapply as needed during the massage. You'll probably find that your bath or shower water extends the life of the oil, allowing you to massage longer without needing to apply more. You might also try smoothing massage oil over your lover's dry skin and then lightly splashing him or her with water. The revitalized oil will become incredibly slippery, and the sensation of water on warm, oiled skin is exquisite.

Sensual Massage Strokes

With your partner facing away from you, leaning on the tub wall for support, begin massaging her back with long, deep strokes that begin at her shoulders and end just above her buttocks. Move up to her shoulders and neck, gently kneading out any tension. Use your body weight for deeper kneading.

As you feel your partner begin to relax, use a lighter touch, focusing on the sensitive areas around the waist and armpit. Using a light, rhythmic touch, interchange long, gliding caresses with shorter, deeper strokes. Move on to the elbows, arms, and hands, and progress down the hips to the legs and feet, brushing the buttocks as you move up and down your partner's body.

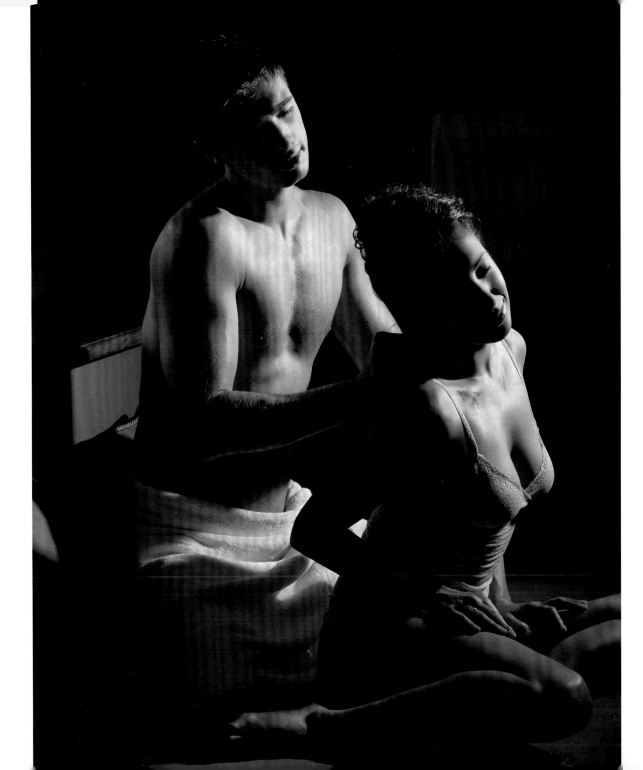

Ask your partner to turn around and lean against the tub wall. Using the same light, rhythmic touch, stroke your partner's chest, arms, and hands. Pay special attention to her breasts, gently stroking and cupping them. His nipples will enjoy attention, too.

Glide down over the belly and hips to your partner's legs, brushing the inner thighs on your way down. Pick up and massage each foot. As you work your way back up your partner's body, tease him or her by brushing the inner thighs again, nearing the pubic triangle, but never quite touching it. Spend more time stroking the belly, waist, and hips, reaching around to cup and stroke the buttocks.

As the erotic energy builds, you and your partner will naturally become ready for some lovemaking. At this point, you can either dry off and take it to the bedroom, or stay wet and finish up in the shower.

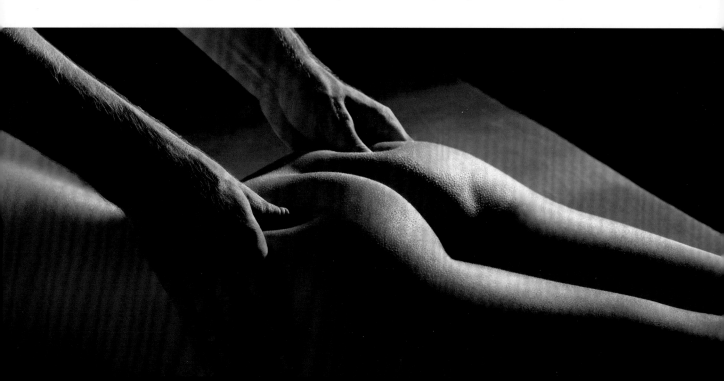

Tub Tantra

The complex spiritual practice of Tantra was first developed over 6,000 years ago in India. Originally a form of protest against religious restrictions on sex, Tantra's core principles encourage practitioners to slow down and enjoy the journey, rather than rushing to climax. Tantra is a dance, without a beginning or end. Benefits of Tantric practice can include enhanced physical health, expanded consciousness, and greater intimacy.

- Begin your practice with the same ritual, something simple like undressing one another, or running the bath, or some other personal task that requires you to do something loving for your partner.

- Wash each other with loving care, being sure to soap and rinse every inch of each other's bodies.

- The man sits in the tub, his legs in front of him—you can also sit on a bathmat next to the tub—and the woman faces him and lowers herself onto him, wrapping her legs around his back and embracing him. This basic Tantra position will allow you to experience each other's bodies and minds simultaneously.

- Listen to each other's breathing. As you inhale and exhale together, your pace will naturally even out, until you are breathing in unison. Try to maintain this harmonious breath throughout your lovemaking.

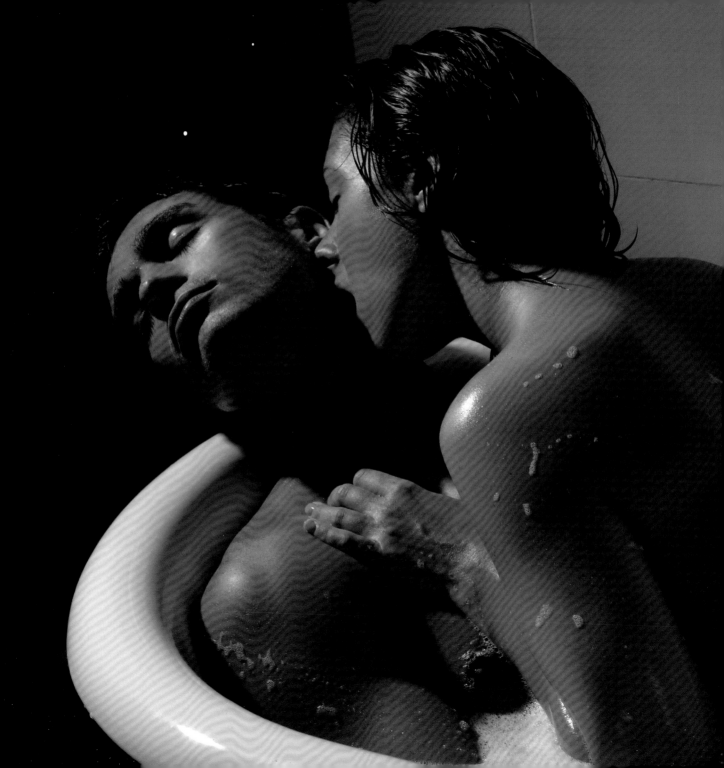

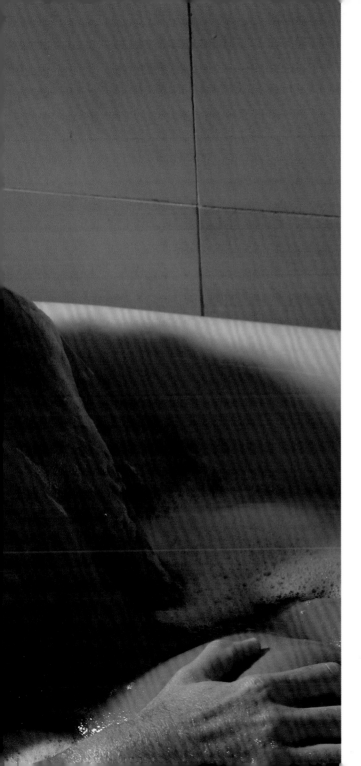

HAPPY ENDINGS

IF YOU AND YOUR PARTNER choose to remain in the tub for your lovemaking, you will soon have to decide how you want to climax!

While of course sex doesn't have to culminate with an orgasm to feel good, there are certain manual techniques that will help you along in this journey, if you so desire.

Manually Pleasuring Him

Apply about a tablespoon of waterproof lube to the palm of your hand and rub it gently over your lover's penis and scrotum. Begin stroking his penis, using the moves outlined in Chapter 6, "The Solo Sensual Bath." Let one goal guide you: prolonging his orgasm as long as possible, which should result in a more powerful climax.

As you stroke his penis and fondle his scrotum, slow down or change what you are doing if ejaculation seems imminent. Vary your technique at the beginning, and then concentrate on one type of stroke, moving faster and harder as he nears orgasm. When you are ready to let him orgasm, you can insert a finger into his rectum and apply pressure to his prostate, guaranteeing explosive results.

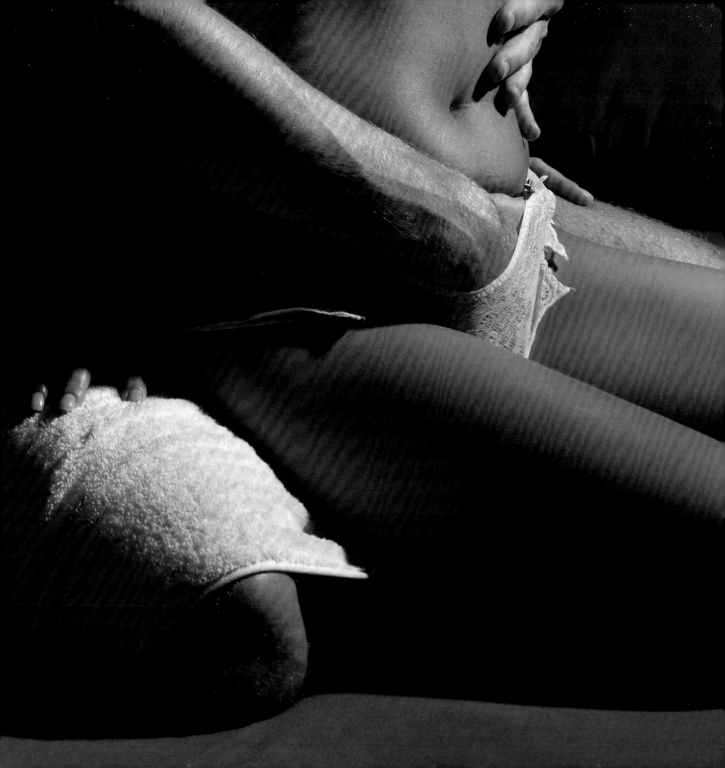

Manually Pleasuring Her

After moistening your fingers with waterproof lube, begin by gently rubbing her entire vulva. As she becomes more aroused, she'll begin to spread her legs a little. Take this as an invitation to explore further and slip a finger between her labia to lightly touch her clitoris, circling it gently. Insert a finger into her vagina and press her G-spot.

Pay close attention to her breathing and to her body's response to your touch. If you find she responds best to G-spot stimulation, apply more pressure. If penetration gets her hot, insert two or three fingers to bring her to orgasm. Most women, however, will respond most visibly to direct clitoral stimulation.

As she nears orgasm, focus on whichever touch pleases her best and continue until she has finished climaxing.

Different Strokes for Her Pleasure

When giving your lover manual pleasure, mix things up with a few different strokes she may not have tried:

- *Spelling*: Use your index finger to trace the alphabet on your lover's clitoris. A good move to begin with, spelling will bring her to a heightened state of arousal.

- *Circling*: With your forefinger and middle finger, rub the clitoris with a gentle, circular motion, varying speed and intensity.
- *Tapping*: Use one finger to gently tap your partner's clitoris, varying the tempo and speed.
- *Drawing*: Use one or two fingers to draw a circle around your partner's clitoris until she begs you for more. This is a good move to combine with tapping.
- *Rolling*: Place your thumb and forefinger on either side of her clitoris and gently roll it between your fingers. Begin with a slow, light roll, and then gradually accelerate the movement until you find the speed that works for her.

As you touch your partner, pay attention to her body language. She may prefer a consistent touch that brings her to orgasm, or she may want you to interchange several different moves.

Tongue Tricks

Although most men love any oral attention they receive, surprise your lover with a few smooth moves that will take his breath away.

- Hold the head of his penis in your mouth, closing your lips around the shaft below it. Use your tongue to trace patterns on the sensitive skin of his glans.

- Take as much of him in your mouth as is comfortable for you, and then gently suck, increasing the pressure and suction gradually.

- Make a circle around his shaft with your thumb and forefinger. Gently glide your fingers up and down the length of him while you flick the head of his penis with the tip of your tongue.

- Pretend his penis is lipstick and trace him over your lips while you look up at him through your eyelashes. This move is guaranteed to drive him wild.

ORAL SEX

PERHAPS THE MOST INTIMATE sexual act, oral sex in the tub can be sublime. Although you might have to work a little bit harder to find the position that works best for both of you, the payoff can be huge. As the steamy room and hot water break down your inhibitions—and soap and water wash away any unpleasant scents and tastes—you may find yourself pleasing your lover in ways that never seemed possible in the bedroom.

Fellatio Fun in the Tub

Before you begin, find a comfortable position that works for both of you. Have him lean against the tub wall while you sit on the edge of the tub, facing him. Recline in the tub while he kneels in front of you, straddling your body. If you have a chair or chaise in your bathroom, make use of it.

Fill your mouth with saliva—or use a waterproof lubricant—and take him into your mouth, wetting the length of his penis. Use one hand to spread the moisture evenly over the length of him and the other hand to fondle or cup his testicles. Holding the base of his penis, flick your tongue over the head of his penis, teasing him. Kiss him the length of his shaft, paying special attention to his frenulum, the sensitive tissue below the head of his penis on the outer side.

Spend as much time as possible slowing working him into a frenzy, varying your touches and licks, using both hands to caress his scrotum, hips, buttocks, thighs, and lower belly. If he responds well to a

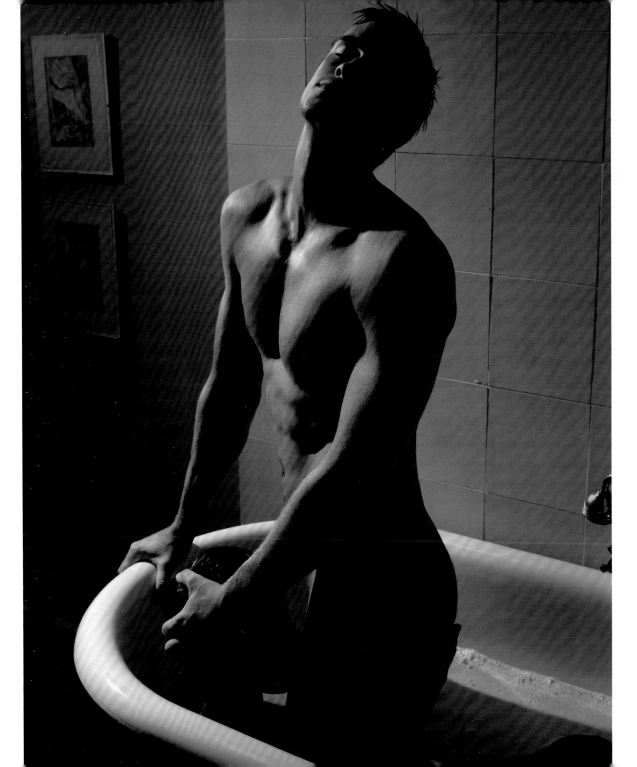

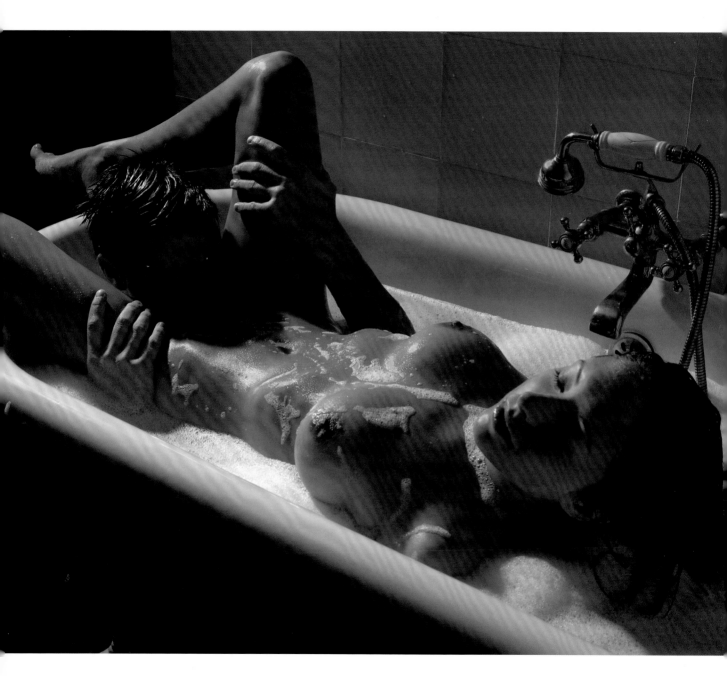

particular sensation, repeat it; if the response is lackluster, move on to something new. Your goal is to prolong his orgasm so that it will be more intense when he does climax. Try to bring him to the brink of pleasure, and then stop, delaying him and prolonging his ecstasy.

As his breath becomes ragged or strained and his thrusting becomes more rhythmic, caress his testicles with one hand and wrap the other around the base of his penis, so that you can comfortably stroke him from the bottom to the middle of his penis. At the same time, use your mouth to pleasure the top half of his penis. As you stroke, lick, and suck simultaneously, he should become more erect. Speed up the pace until he climaxes.

Keep in mind that oral sex should be about the journey, not the destination. If either of you have problems climaxing, move on to something else. Oral sex feels good, with or without an orgasm at the end of it. Take pleasure in the pleasure you are giving or receiving, and try not to worry about who comes first.

Tub-time Cunnilingus

Before you begin to pleasure her orally, fill your mouth with saliva so your mouth isn't dry when you're performing cunnilingus, which can be uncomfortable for your partner. After you have kissed, stroked, and licked the area around her vagina, gently spread her pubic lips, revealing her clitoris. Don't attack her love button—be gentle with her clitoris until she directs otherwise.

As she breathes faster and tenses her body, increase your pace and intensity, varying the way you lick her vulva, labia, clitoris, and vaginal opening. When she indicates you're doing something she likes, keep at it until she relaxes again. Try not to hold back the clitoral hood unless she asks you to; the clitoris is very sensitive, and not every woman enjoys direct stimulation to it. Most women enjoy intense vaginal stimulation up to and through the time they orgasm. Don't stop until she's climaxed.

While you're performing oral sex on her, try a couple of "fancy" moves, sure to get her attention and give her pleasure:

- Trace the alphabet on her clitoris with your tongue. Because this move doesn't usually lead directly to orgasm, this is a good technique to use toward the beginning of your oral play.
- Circle her clitoris with just the tip of your tongue, applying a light, direct touch until she screams for more.
- Insert your tongue into her vagina during oral sex, moving it in large circles while inside her.

When you repeat the same motion too much, she can become desensitized to it, so vary your technique until she builds to an orgasm.

If your partner is amenable, incorporate anal play into your oral lovemaking. Many women enjoy anilingus, also known as rimming, but allow her to set the pace. When you sense she is getting ready to climax, insert a finger into her rectum. Sometimes this small "nudge" will send her over the edge.

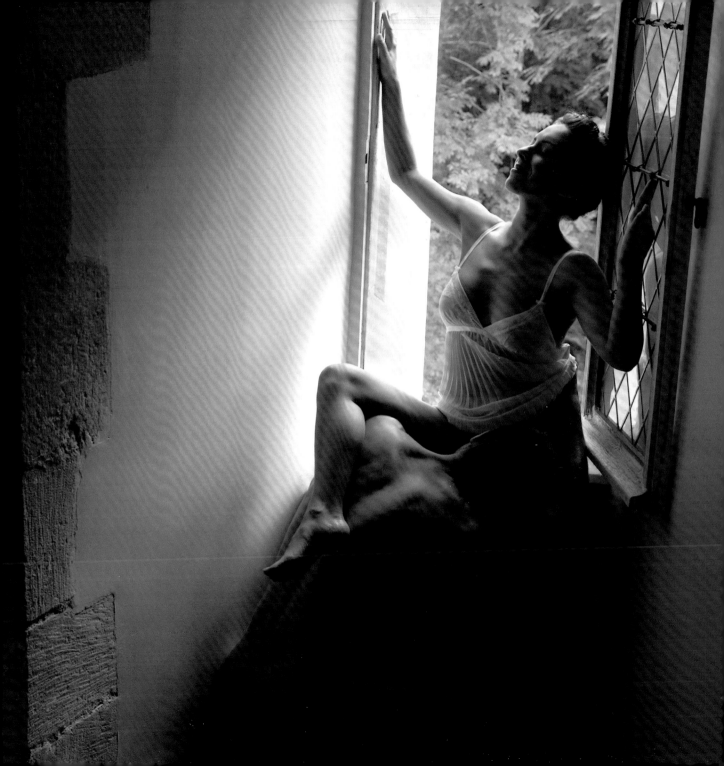

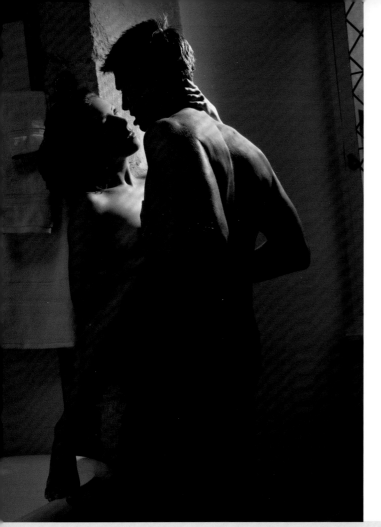

INTERCOURSE

MANY COUPLES ENJOY heading straight for sex, while others like to detour into manual or oral pleasure along the way. No matter your route, if you arrive at penetration, you'll want to keep a few things in mind if you're going to do it in the shower.

First and foremost, always use lubricant. Hot water dehydrates the flesh and washes away natural lubrication. Choose a silicone-based lube, and use plenty of it. You'll find that even if you step outside the shower's spray and dry off a bit, a sprinkle of fresh water will reactivate the lubricant.

The bathtub and shower can be hard on soft flesh, so try not to get too rough so you don't slip and seriously injure yourself or your partner. If you decide sex in the tub is something you'd like to do often, consider installing a handrail and applying nonstick decals to the floor of the tub.

Dripping wet and glistening with scented oil, my lover's body and mine slap together rhythmically as we meet under the warm shower spray. My lover holds my hands above my head and turns me, so that I face the shower wall, before engaging me again from behind.

—*Tara, 34*

Tub-friendly Sex Positions

Unless you are fortunate enough to have an extra-large tub, you'll probably find the missionary position isn't the most comfortable pick for a sensual bath. Spice up your lovemaking using one—or more!—of these bathtub-friendly positions.

Kneeling, Man Behind

The woman kneels in the tub, facing the tub wall, while the man kneels behind her, taking her from behind. Many couples will have experimented with "doggie style" sex in bed, so this is another good beginner's position.

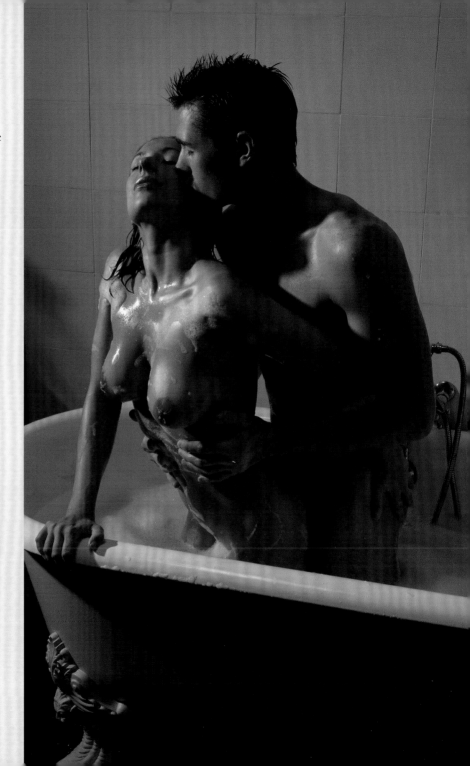

Woman on Top

The man sits in a partially filled tub, reclining against the tub wall, while the woman lowers herself onto his penis, straddles him, and wraps her legs around his torso. Ironically, this position gives the man control of most of the movement. If the woman wants to take charge, she can kneel in the same position, or use her legs to push off the tub wall.

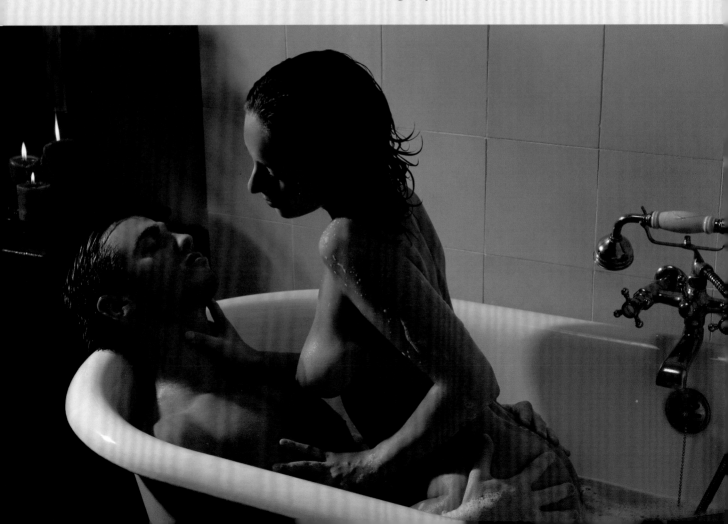

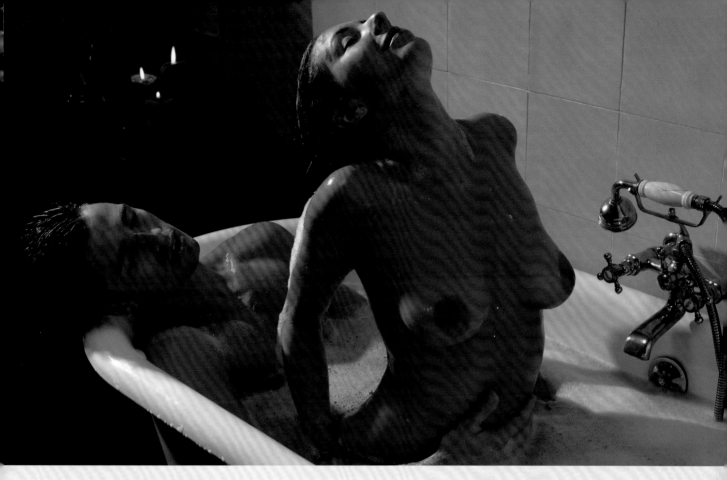

Reverse Cowgirl

The man sits in the middle of the tub, leaning against the tub wall, and the woman lowers herself onto him, with her back to his front. In this position, the woman will have limited movement, so the man will need to hold her around the waist or, if she's tall enough, she can thrust by pushing off from the opposite tub wall. This variation on "doggie style" sex gives the man lots of opportunities to caress the woman's breasts and clitoris, so "Lap Sitting" is a good position for women who need extra stimulation in order to reach orgasm.

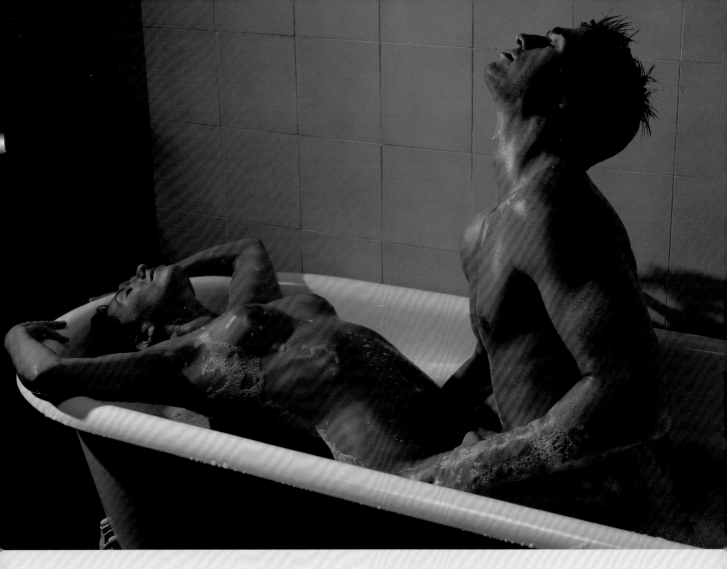

Legs Up

The man kneels in the middle of the tub while the woman sits and reclines against the tub wall. With the woman holding the edges of the tub for support, the man lifts her legs, wraps them around his waist and thrusts gently into her.

Standing, Man Behind

The woman stands, facing the wall and using the tub wall or safety bar for support, while the man engages her from behind. Another intimate variation on "doggie style" sex, "Standing, Man Behind" allows the man to caress the woman's curves during lovemaking.

Tub-time Tips

WATERPROOF KNEEPADS

For any position that involves kneeling in the tub, slip a folded washcloth or hand towel under each knee. You'll notice improved traction, and your knees won't be sore when the fun is done.

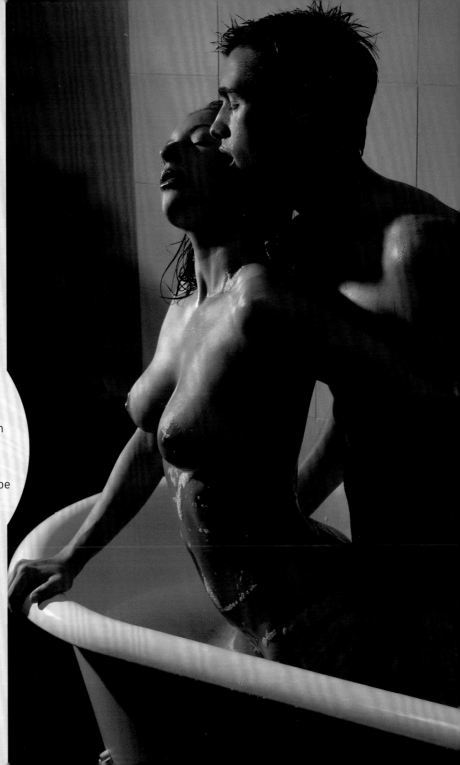

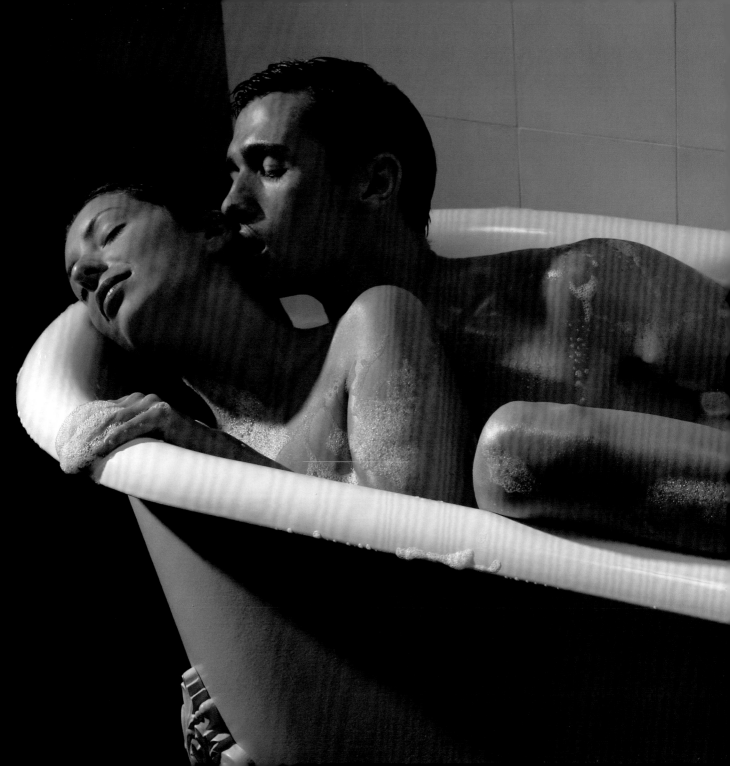

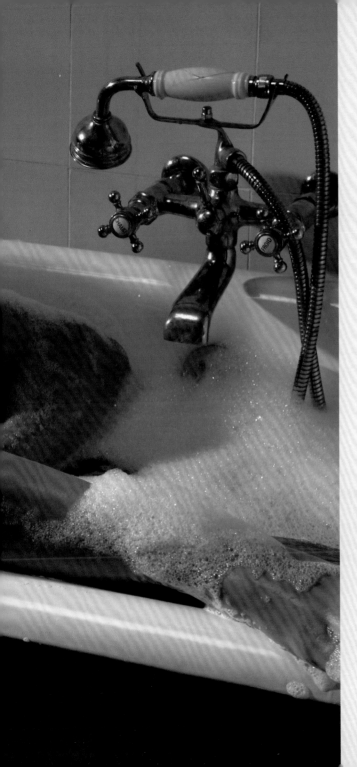

Butterfly

The man and woman curl into the tub, both facing the same direction, as if they were spooning, while the man takes her from behind. This position will only work if both partners fit comfortably in the tub, if your tub is big enough, or if you and your partner are small enough, you'll both find this position sensual and intimate.

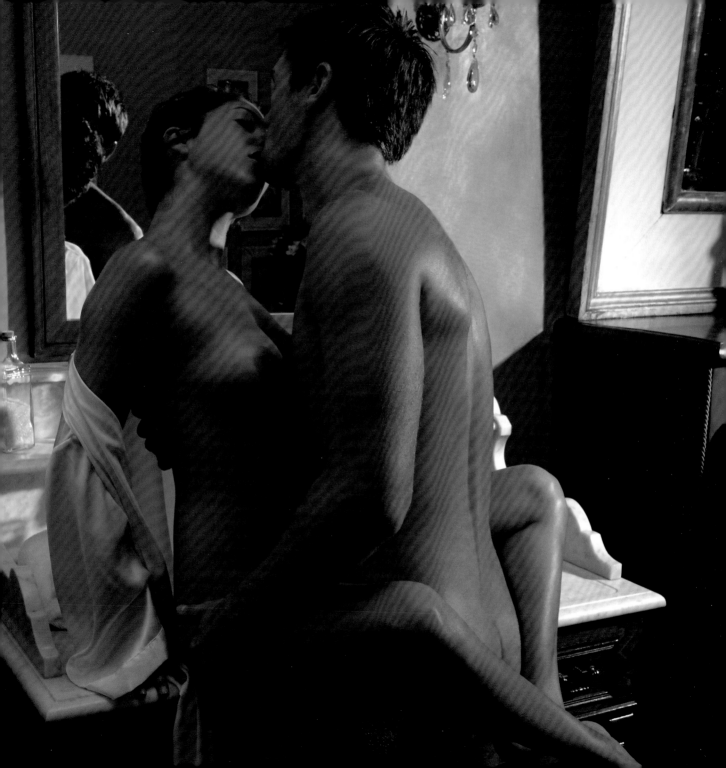

Standing and Carrying

The man stands in the tub (you can also lean against a sink to get started!), leaning against the wall for support, while the woman faces him. After standing on the tub edge, using the wall or safety bar for support, the woman lowers herself onto the man's penis and he lifts her legs over his arms. This position sounds complicated, but it affords deep penetration.

Using Toys During Intercourse

Sex toys aren't just for foreplay! If she has trouble climaxing during penetration, use a clitoral vibrator to tickle her fancy while you're making love. Some remote-controlled waterproof vibrators have been designed for use during vaginal sex. She slips on the "panties," and you hold the remote. Another great couple's toy is the waterproof vibrating erection ring, which fits over the base of his penis. A built-in clitoral vibrator buzzes her clitoris and stimulates her G-spot.

I've always loved bathing, so bringing my lover into the tub with me was a natural progression in my relationship with John. Our ritual begins when we settle into the tub, my back against his chest, and he lathers me up and massages my shoulders and breasts. The feeling of his soapy, slippery hands is very exciting. Not only does it prepare us for a long night of lovemaking, but also the intimacy we share in the bath brings us closer together as a couple.

—Suzy, 35

BASKING IN THE AFTERGLOW

AFTER YOUR PLAY HAS ENDED, take a few
moments to enjoy the relaxing and invigorating effects
of your time together in the bath. Gently dry one
another off with clean, plush bath sheets. With a
fragrant, rich moisturizing cream, moisturize each
other's skin, locking in moisture and sealing the
intimate bond you've formed in the tub.

Before you reenter the world of children and
mortgages, bills, and "to do" lists and your jobs,
acknowledge the experience you and your lover have
just shared together. If possible, retire to bed immediately following your sensual bath, so that the sweetness
of your union can color your dreams.

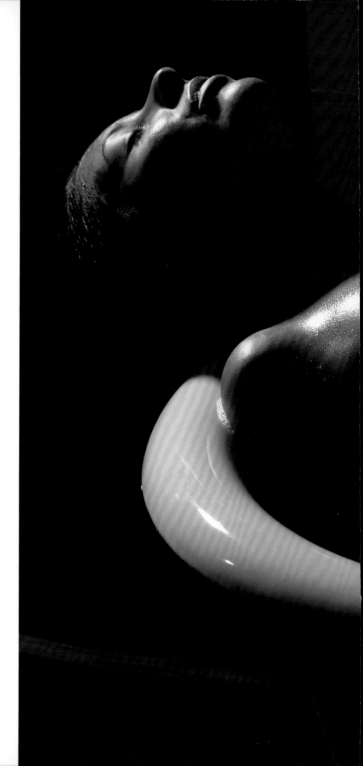

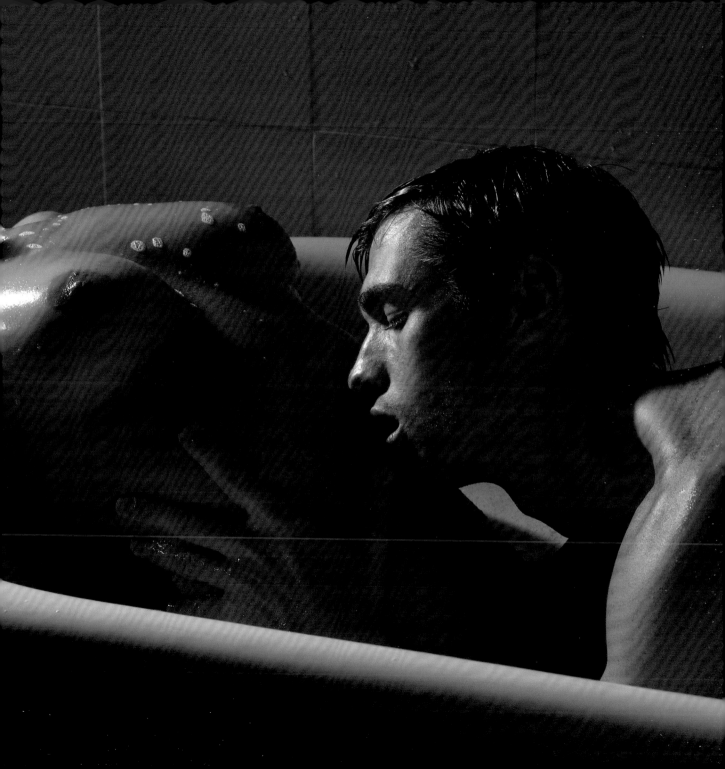

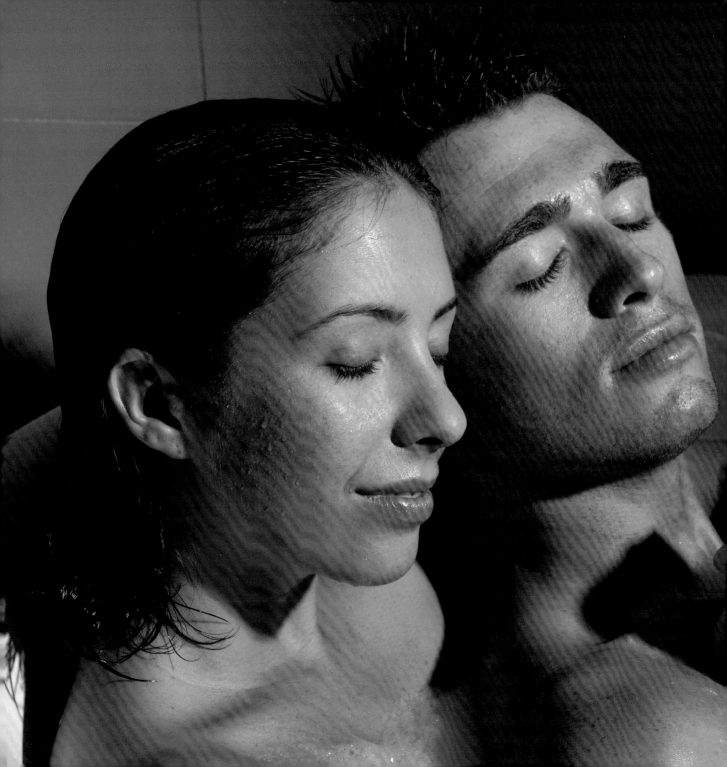

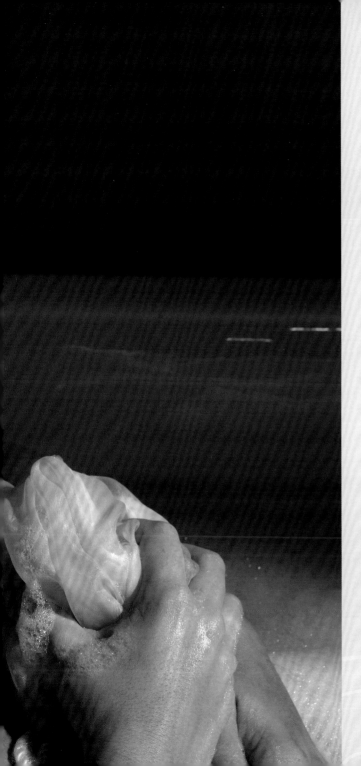

ABOUT THE AUTHOR

TAMAR LOVE is a freelance writer and editor with nine years of professional experience. In addition to authoring the book *Plan a Fabulous Party in No Time*, Tamar spent two years as the staff writer for MyPleasure (www.mypleasure.com), writing most of the e-business's marketing and educational content, including dozens of articles about sexual health and technique. She was also the ghostwriter for About.com's Sexuality channel, authoring dozens of articles and product guides during the three years she managed the Web site. Tamar received her master of arts in creative writing from San Francisco State University in 2000. She lives in Lake Balboa, California, with her husband, cats, and dogs.

Index

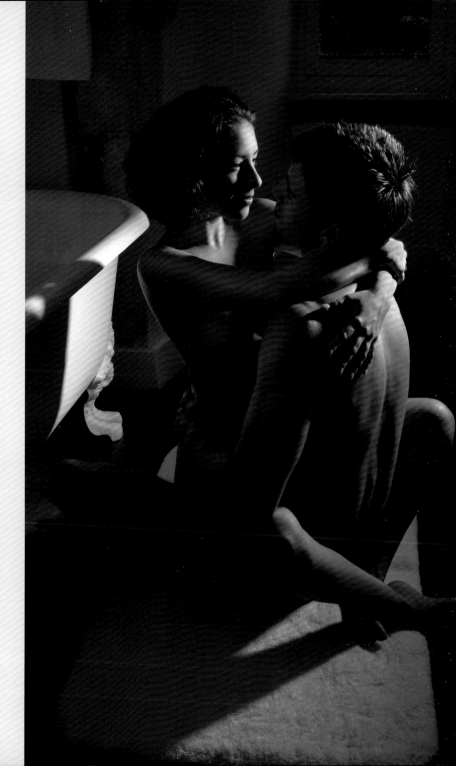

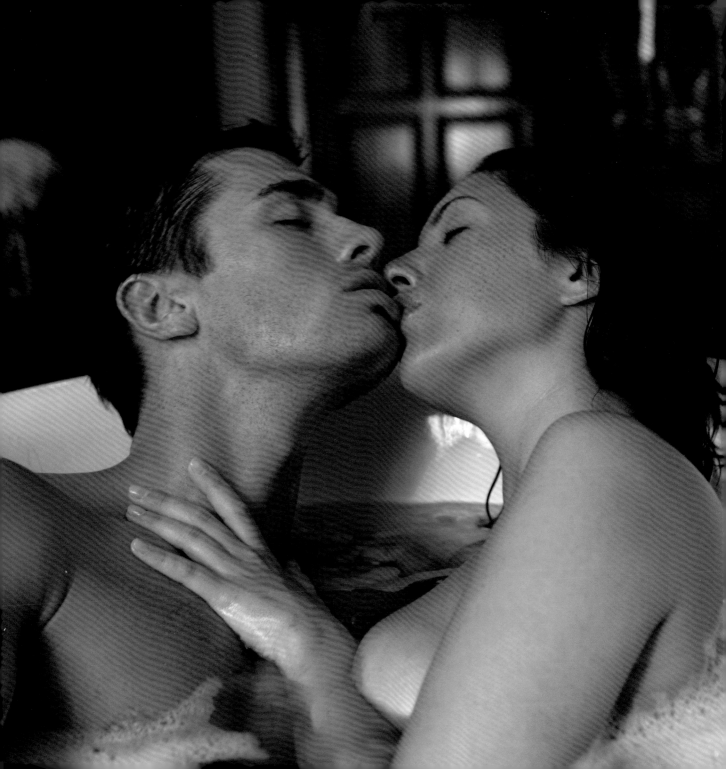